A
Language Program
for the
Nonlanguage Child

Burl B. Gray
Bruce P. Ryan

Research Press   2612 N Mattis   Champaign, Illinois 61820

Portions of the information presented in this book resulted from
research grant OEG-0-9-142144-3554(032) from the Office of Education, Department of Health, Education and Welfare, Washington, D. C.

Copies of this book may be ordered from the publisher at the address
given on the title page.

ISBN 0-87822-034-8

3/8/78 pl· 6·9r

Contents

List of Tables

List of Figures

Foreword

This book was written for students, teachers (clinicians), and researchers. The authors present a behavioral interpretation of language, a
resultant teaching strategy, and data from eight years of experience
with the method. This information is presented in a manner such that
the reader can identify and locate that specific aspect in which he is
interested. The first chapter of the book presents a behavioral description of the critical concepts involved in language training and puts forth
a basic teaching strategy called programmed conditioning. Chapters Two
and Three elaborate upon the basic structure of programmed conditioning and develop a total language training strategy. This includes a
detailed description of the entire teaching protocol. Chapter Four presents the data and findings of eight years of work on programmed
conditioning for language. In this chapter the authors present results of
their work with a cross section of language disorders. In Chapter Five
the authors engage in some philosophical and speculative discussions
about the nature and the development of language. They present a
basic behavioral model to explain the acquisition of language in an
effort to promote critical research in this vital area and suggest some
directions for the future study of language acquisition and training.

Preface

This book is intended for both the college student and the practitioner. It is essentially a report of the conclusions drawn after eight years of effort to develop a universal language training procedure. We have presented our interpretation of the critical issues, illustrated our solution based upon that interpretation, and verified our solution through data.

Language is the essence of human survival. It is the uniqueness of man. Many people have said many things about language, its development, its structure, and its teaching. Unfortunately, some have chosen to influence language teachers through theory rather than with data. Unfortunately, untested linguistic theory frequently persists despite the absence of empirical proof. We have tried to rigorously respond to this mythological pedagogy which has run rampant for so long. We have endeavored to make no suggestion for training which was not supported by empirical test results. We have made an effort to present only a data bound training strategy.

The authors engage in some clearly identified speculation in the last chapter. However, the validity of the training strategy—programmed conditioning—should be determined from the data presented, not from the believability of this indulgence in rhetoric.

Many people have contributed significantly to the work which this book represents. Lily Fygetakis not only helped in the original program planning, but was the first person to use the program. Barbara London and Sue Stancyk also provided valuable information as clinical language teachers who continuously tested new programs and procedures. Many other teachers and volunteers aided and extended this effort. Peers who made frequent visits to our project provided many valuable and critical insights and suggestions. It is these people, who are in fact a part of this book, to whom we dedicate this work.

Monterey, California   B.B.G.
February 1973   B.P.R.

1 Programmed Conditioning: The Instructional Equation

This book has only one purpose: to present a rationale for and a procedure to teach nonlanguage children how to talk. Throughout this book, the word language refers to the ability of a speaker in a novel environment to generate a syntactically correct and situationally appropriate sentence that he has not just previously heard.

Language is an enormously complex and ill-understood topic. The problem of teaching a nonuser how to use the language is even less defined. Since it is easy to devote an entire book to one small aspect of language, we circumscribe our considerations here to one aspect—teaching language. Those questions which we wish to consider must be chosen very carefully. The prime consideration is that they be relevant to the topic of teaching language. In order to differentiate some critical points, we will first briefly consider our understanding of some of the fundamental aspects of language.

The Structure of Language

Language is viewed as the symbolic representation of information which is being transferred from one person to another person(s). Language is the vehicle through which that information is coded, represented, and transferred. If I wish to give you the information that I am hungry, I must code this into some symbolic form which we have in common, and I must display this code to you. The display usually takes the form of talking, writing, gesturing, or some combination of these. The spoken code itself is a structure having phonemic, morphologic, syntactic, and semantic components.

The display (model of transmission) in which we are most interested here is talking. Talking implies the observable use of a verbal code which is mutually understood by sender and recipient. The phonemic and morphological components describe the constraints of the sounds used and the way in which they are clustered (words). The grammatic component describes the temporal ordering of and the relationship between words and classes of words. It represents the rules of usage. The semantic component describes the meaning or intent of the message which is being transferred.

The *act* of talking is an observable performance on the part of the sender. The reception of the message can only be ascertained by observing some consequent *act* (performance) on the part of the receiver. If I display (perform) the code "I am hungry," my only confirmation of the fact that you received it would be some consequent observable performance on your part, such as answering "Me too, let's eat." Any time the performance of the receiver does not confirm his reception of the preceding code we have no information about whether he "actually" received it or not. Receiver confirmation can be either verbal or nonverbal. If it is nonverbal, we may not know if the receiver cannot verbalize the language code or if he can but chooses not to do so. Frequent clinical difficulty is in determining if a silent child can't talk or if he won't talk. On the other hand, if the confirmation is verbal, we know that he did receive the message and that he can use the verbal code to transmit information.

There is a nonverbal aspect of language communication. Facial and body gesturing frequently accompanies verbal language. However, the most frequent problem with nonlanguage children is that they don't talk. Seldom, if ever, do parents complain that a child's verbal language is fine but his gesture language performance is deficient. In fact the situation is usually just the opposite; therefore, we tend to concentrate upon the verbal aspect of language.

People who are concerned about the presence of receptive language often use nonverbal language behavior as evidence of its presence. The speculation here is that a child must have receptive language before expressive language can occur. A behavioral definition of this position is that a child must demonstrate a nonverbal performance in response to verbal statements by others before he is capable of demonstrating verbal performance to those statements. Although this is a frequently observed sequence of appearance in young children, that does not mean that it is a compulsory sequence for development nor a mandatory sequence for instructional purposes. Certainly the behavior of people is frequently the opposite. Most adults, as well as children, will have a verbal language performance for flying airplanes prior to their nonverbal performance, i.e., flying an airplane. To make the supposition that one *must* have a nonverbal performance before he can have a verbal performance is to argue that one must fly an airplane before he can talk about flying an airplane. This argues against common experience as well as research findings (Berko, 1958; Guess, et al., 1968; Gray and Fygetakis, 1968a; Guess, 1969).

In a study of this point, Guess (1969) trained two subjects in receptive (pointing) behavior for singular-plural morpheme discrimination. Following that phase he then trained them in the productive counterpart of the first training. In the third phase he trained the subjects to respond to the receptive behavior task again, but this time he reversed the rule, i.e., pointing to a singular item when a plural name is given. During these various training phases Guess occasionally probed for correct usage of the verbal component. He found that productive speech did not follow automatically from a demonstration of receptive ability. Also, he found that after productive speech was established a reversal in the receptive performance rules and the receptive performance itself did not cause the productive or verbal behavior to similarly reverse. His findings led him to conclude "that receptive language and expressive speech can be two separate and functionally independent classes of behavior" (Guess, 1969, p. 63).

Although others (Myklebust, 1957; McCarthy, 1954; Lee, 1970) tend to place considerable importance upon receptive (nonverbal) performance as a prerequisite to verbal performance the weight of the evidence and data appears to suggest otherwise. Although we will consider the presence of both nonverbal and verbal performance as being critical to complete language adequacy, we will not make the instructional constraint that the nonverbal performance must be taught (appear) before the verbal performance can be acquired.

Normal Language Acquisition

Almost every discussion of language at some time or other deals with what is called normal language acquisition or normal language development. This refers to the manner in which normal speakers become users of the language. There are two primary aspects to normal language acquisition: the first is that process by which one becomes able to use the language; the second is the temporal sequence in which various language forms appear.

With respect to the question of how language develops, there are two major schools of thought. People of a psycholinguistic persuasion (Chomsky, 1965, 1966; Lenneberg, 1969; Fodor and Katz, 1964; McNeill, 1966, 1968; Jacobovits and Miron, 1967; Dixon and Horton, 1968; Smith and Miller, 1966) argue that the development of language is a natural process which is psychobiophysically dictated through the language acquisition device. Others (Skinner, 1957; Lovaas, 1968; Sloane and MacAulay, 1968; Guess, 1968; Sulzbacher and Costello, 1970; Gray, 1969) support the position that language is a learned phenomenon and can be accounted for by principles of learning. The argument becomes quite detailed and is more fully explored in other literature (Chomsky, 1967 a and b; Jacobovits and Miron, 1967; Guess, 1969; Gray, 1969, 1970).

For our present concern of teaching language, this currently popular question about normal language acquisition is not particularly relevant. The critical question is not whether or not normal language development happens because of learning principles; but rather, can language be taught to nonusers via principles of learning? If we assume that the appearance of language is determined by some maturational template of the organism, then we must ask—as Englemann (1970) did—if this means that we should give up on a nonlanguage child and just wait for him to mature?

The developmental philosophy implies there is a fixed order of occurrence of language subcomponents. From this frame of reference a child cannot produce verbal language until all of the preceding subcomponents are present. That is, he cannot use verbal language until he is developmentally ready. Once again, we refer to Englemann for a concise view on readiness.

> The notion of readiness is based upon the developmental assumption that something magical happens to a child with age. From the teaching-oriented view, nothing magical can happen. The child is simply taught concepts. The longer the period of time, the more concepts he is taught. Unless the child's performance is expressed in these terms, there is no remedy for the child who is not ready except to let time exert its magical influence on his development (Englemann, 1970, p. 115).

Interestingly enough, the fact that language training is sought for children and the fact that the teaching of language has become such a social priority confirms the view that the developmental philosophy has been found wanting. Every nonlanguage child is a walking refutation of the idea of innate natural language development. By definition, candidates for language training are children (or sometimes adults) who failed to develop it normally. The magical influence of the passage of time has not produced it. The alternative then is to teach it. For the language teacher there is no other alternative. Even those teachers who ascribe to the developmental philosophy of language acquisition must end up *teaching* language. There is no way they can go inside the child and alter the developmental biology in a prescribed manner to cause language to begin to develop.

In all of this the critical element is that the validity of a teaching procedure can be tested. The outcome of our teaching will reflect upon the soundness of our original logic and our procedures. And the success, or lack of it, may be construed to have some bearing upon the hypotheses of normal acquisition.

The second aspect of normal language acquisition— the temporal sequence in which the various language forms appear— does have a more direct bearing upon language training. This information becomes important from two standpoints. First, it is possible to construct normative profiles, i.e., language proficiency tests. These tests can provide information about the degree of language ability for a given child. The necessity for and the urgency of training can be based to some extent upon the performance of a child on such a test. Two notable examples of this type of utilization of normal language acquisition information are Lee (1970) and Lillywhite, et al. (1970).

The second important use of this temporal sequence data is in maximizing the probability of success in language training. Although it is possible to teach language forms without following such a temporal sequence (Gray and Fygetakis, 1968 a, b; Guess, et al.,1968; Guess, 1969), it would appear likely that the task might be made easier by doing so. It is doubtful if a sequence of developmental usage exists in the normal environment which is totally without functional advantage for the user. Therefore, a teaching strategy should capitalize upon this information insofar as it is practical and useful and does not conflict with any constraints of the teaching plan.

It is very important to be fully aware of these two different aspects of normal language acquisition. A question about normal language acquisition is valid only if it is relevant to the problem of teaching language.

The Nonlanguage Child

A more apt definition of a nonlanguage child is a nonperformer of the verbal-linguistic code. He most generally has some type of nonverbal language which may be grammatical under special rules of gesture language. A distinctive trait about the child is that, despite growing up in a verbal-linguistic environment, he fails to perform verbally himself. The complaint is that all code sending and confirmation of reception is nonverbal—or if verbal, it violates syntactic rules of usage. Specifically, the verbal-linguistic performance of the child is not appropriate. It makes no difference what label is assigned to the fact of nonperformance (autistic, receptive aphasic, dysphasic, language delayed, brain damaged, etc.), the teaching job is still the same. The language teacher must *change* the child's code sending *performance*. All judgment about the adequacy of language ability must ultimately be based upon some *performance* on the part of the user. Giving a name to the reason why we think he has not begun to use the language in no way alters the teaching task, in *all* cases the job is to teach language.

It might appear that we are insensitive to the quite obvious differences that exist between the various categories of nonperformance listed above, such as autistic, hard of hearing, etc. We have all heard that no two children are alike and that as teachers we must respond to the individual differences of each student; however, the task is one of becoming selectively responsive to individual differences that are meaningful in terms of the teaching strategy. To indiscriminately respond to all observable differences is to invite failure.

Individual differences which specifically jeopardize a student's capacity to perform in the teaching situation should be dealt with: if he is hard of hearing, we must use amplification; if he is big for his age, we might have to find a larger chair and desk; etc. These types of alterations, while very important to the student's success with the procedure, do not represent gross changes in any basic instructional strategy. If a totally new strategy must be designed for each student or for each individual difference, the job soon becomes impossible.

This problem can be overcome if we remember that effective teaching strategies depend upon universal characteristics which are shared by prospective students as well as upon their individual differences. Specifically, all language nonperformers have important characteristics in common: first, they don't use the language; second, they all learn behavior according to the same general principles as we currently understand them. The teaching strategy must be based upon these types of universals. Individual differences should be responded to if—and only if, they constitute a threat to the success of the child while he is operating on these universals. The universals define the basic strategy. The individual differences dictate the adjustments that will be necessary in that strategy in order to fine tune it for a given student.

The Philosophy of Evaluation

It is important now to consider the influence of the diagnostic activity on the area of language teaching. The underlying philosophy of the diagnostic examiner sets the stage for the entire training process. The examiner decides what information will be sought and, just as importantly, what information will *not* be sought. This selection process colors the teaching activity that will follow; therefore, it is very important that the examiner have a philosophy and an orientation that is complimentary to those of the teaching procedure.

When a language teacher (clinician) is preparing to teach a nonlanguage child language, certain critical information must be obtained. A plan for teaching must be developed. What should the child be asked to do? What should the teacher do? How should it be done? Answers to these questions provide the strategy. Without this information and planning, the teaching (learning) time is spent unproductively and with no direction.

Thus, the one most important event of teaching language is deciding upon the strategy to be used. In order to arrive at a plan the teacher must have specific information; therefore, the clinical purpose for a "diagnostic session" is to obtain that information. The knowledge a clinician has about a child and his language is determined by the questions that are asked. If considerable diagnostic effort is spent obtaining information, it will be used presumably in the formulation of the teaching plan.

Any diagnostic battery should, in the ideal sense, reduce the number of clinical options that are potentially available to the teacher to one. Therefore, any question whose answer does not reduce the clinical options is not related to the task and should be replaced.

Just as clinical strategy information is obtained from the questions, the questions themselves are determined by the prevailing philosophy of the examiner, typically based upon the medical model. Its major premise is that behavior is a symptom or outward sign of a deeper underlying problem or disease, whose successful treatment must focus upon the underlying cause. When applied to language, it presumes that no teaching can be successfully accomplished until the original cause has been determined. This model generates a line of diagnostic interrogation which includes extensive case history information on items pertaining to the pre- and post-natal periods as well as subsequent medical-development information including: the duration of the mother's labor, birth weight, use of forceps during delivery, sibling order, age child sat alone, age child walked, high fevers, etc. Unless clinical options are available which are responsive to conditions such as birth weight, duration of labor, etc., it is difficult to see any relationship between the information obtained and its intended use in formulating a teaching strategy for language (Englemann, 1970).

The problem is that the child "doesn't talk much." He does not *do* something that others think he should be *doing*. Historical information about the child may permit, or even encourage, a speculation about why the child did not learn language originally (Wyatt, 1969). In fact, that may be its only purpose. This type of information does not give a teacher many clues about how to teach him language. The practical futility of overemphasis on diagnostic questions which are not tied to specific clinical options is that, after gathering all that information, the child still is not *doing* something and the teacher has gained very little information about what to teach or how to teach him to *do* it.

The functional clinical questions to be answered are (a) What does the child do (or not do) now?, and (b) What should the child be doing? Clinical strategy must answer the question of how to get from a to b. If the philosophical model of interrogation provides us with inappropriate questions and useless answers, we should look for a more appropriate set of operational procedures to help in the construction of a strategy for language training.

Programmed Conditioning: An Alternative

The educational process assumes language, it does not teach it. The teaching model uses language for information transfer. Thus, the non-language child faces educational disenfranchisement in addition to the other problems commensurate with the lack of language. The problem is one of devising an instructional strategy for teaching language to nonlanguage children.

Any such training strategy should be both as successful and as rapid as possible. The need for success and for economy of time is particularly pointed in language training for young children. Any efficient training strategy which maximizes these values can be described in terms of two major areas: the delivery system and the information load. The delivery system is essentially the coordination and execution of the specific teaching strategy used. The information load is that class of behaviors which is being taught.

The Delivery System

One of the basic considerations in such an instructional equation is the deliberate and correct use of information about human learning. The literature of behavior modification presents a learning theory rationale for the change and control of human behavior in addition to a wide variety of procedures for achieving the desired behavior. The efficacy of teaching strategies which deliberately adhere to principles of learning is quite well substantiated in the literature and does not need review here (Yates, 1970; Ayllon and Azrin, 1968; Bandura, 1969; Eysenck, 1960; Krasner and Ullman, 1965; Wolpe, 1958). Based upon this evidence, it would appear that any attempt at designing a high precision teaching strategy must incorporate the critical elements of the learning process. In fact, there is doubt if it is possible to avoid it. At the moment the only choice appears to be whether or not to go about it in a systematic way (Meyerson, 1971).

The basic learning sequence is *conditioning*. Within this framework, the conditioning process is viewed in terms of Stimulus-Response-Consequence. The consequence of a response has the potential to either accelerate or decelerate the frequency of future occurrences of that response (Ayllon and Azrin, 1968). Decelerators are often called punishers and accelerators are termed reinforcers. The notation for a reinforcer is S+. Figure 1 highlights the relationships of these three primary units of the learning process.

Figure 1   **Schematic Representation of the Three Primary Elements of the Learning Process**

CONDITIONING

Stimulus ──────────→ Response ──────────→ Stimulus^{+}

Controlled presentation of either or both of the first and third elements of this sequence by another person for the purpose of changing the response is *teaching*, and the person exercising that control is a teacher.

Figure 2   Schematic Representation of the Concept
            of Programming

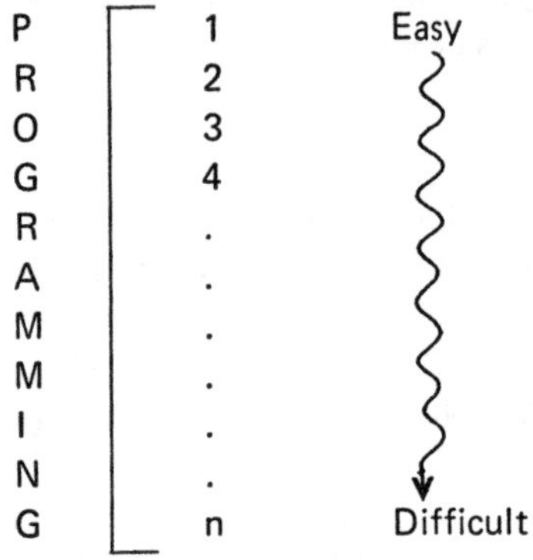

P   1   Easy
R   2
O   3
G   4
R   .
A   .
M   .
M   .
I   .
N   .
G   n   Difficult

Numerous examples of the effectiveness of this approach have been published as noted previously in this chapter.

Studies in psychology and education have found that the teaching process can be speeded up if the learning task proceeds logically and sequentially in small steps from the easier to the more difficult levels of response complexity. This progression is termed programming (Pipe, 1966), and represents one of the most sophisticated methods for the organization and pacing of educational materials (Skinner, 1958; Hendershot, 1964; Pipe, 1966).

Generally, it may be said that with conditioning procedures we have highly efficient techniques for modifying and/or "implanting" specific behavior; and with programming we have a highly organized structure which can pace and co-ordinate teaching activities and material.

The plan would be to "fit" the highly efficient conditioning techniques into an organizational structure (programming) which would closely co-ordinate each response with every other response to be conditioned. If this were achieved, it might be possible to create a maximal learning situation wherein the child would be able to select those cues necessary to construct the language system.

Figure 3

Figure 3 **Schematic Representation of Programmed Conditioning**

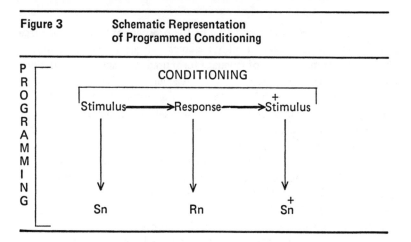

This particular strategy is *programmed conditioning.* The Stimulus-Response-Consequation sequence is arranged such that successive steps will take the behavior in question from its current level to a point where we want it to be. The effort will be to systematically change the S-R-S+ to advance from a basic form of the response to a target performance level.

The Information Load

If programmed conditioning is the training strategy to be used, the first variable to be specified is the response sequence and the content information to be loaded into our delivery system will be language.

Figure 4 **Specification of the Information Load for the Delivery System (Programmed Conditioning)**

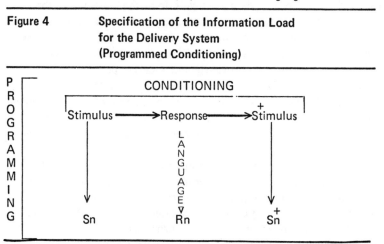

Brief introspection on the prospect of teaching language usage to a potential speaker quickly becomes a staggering impossibility. The possible combinations of language form usage and speaking situations appear to be virtually endless. Thus, the teacher must give the potential user a basic competence in handling an infinite system. One rational way of doing this is in discovering the universal rules which must be known in order to account for all correct combinations of forms and situations. Grammar, of course, is the key.

Although linguists differ among themselves concerning the various aspects of language structure (Fodor and Katz, 1964; Dixon and Horton, 1968), there is sufficient agreement on the general principles (Lee, 1966; Menyuk, 1969) to permit a language teacher to respond to some universals of the teaching procedure.

Criticism is occasionally voiced against linguists because their literature gives the reader no information on how to teach language. It only describes the language structure. In this case it must be remembered that linguists are not being asked to define a teaching protocol, but rather they are being asked to indicate which aspects of the language should be taught. It is appropriate to present this situation to them.

Whenever conditioning techniques are considered as a method for language acquisition in nonlanguage or linguistically divergent children, there is a tendency to focus attention upon conditioning into the behavior a group of verbal responses which have an immediate value to the child socially and environmentally. From the survival point of view this would appear to be both logical and practical. This approach can be described as considering the word to be the basic unit of the language. The majority of these words can be called *content words*, i.e., words which have concrete referents. The other general class of words, *function words*, is often passed over. Function words do not have independent referents but provide grammatical context for the content words (Lee, 1966). Examples of function words include articles, prepositions, auxiliary verbs, etc. This class of words and the rules represented can only be demonstrated in sentences, therefore, an approach to teaching which emphasizes grammar must consider the sentence as the basic linguistic unit.

The neglect of function words and grammar will result in a child who responds to certain situations with a predictable and stereotyped verbal response often described as telegraphic speech. The result is not propositional language (Menyuk, 1964, 1969; Lenneberg, 1969), but one in which the more prominent characteristics of the teaching approach views the word as the basic linguistic teaching unit. The ability of conditioning procedures to effect this type of behavior is rather common in the literature (Lovaas, 1968; Sloane and MacAulay, 1968). Indeed normal language development does appear to begin with the acquisition and use of a corpus of content words (Lillywhite, et al., 1970; Menyuk, 1969; Lee, 1970; Lenneberg, 1964; Wyatt, 1969). However, if only content words are learned to the exclusion of function words, then grammatical language will not develop. The current procedures, while dealing with both the morphology and the grammar, will emphasize grammar and its development. Grammar represents the universal rules by which the user can handle the seemingly infinite series of language productions.

Quite obviously, any meaningful attempt to teach language must handle phonology and morphology as well as grammar. It is interesting to note that it is possible to teach both the phonology and/or the morphology of a language without teaching its grammar (Guess, 1969; Guess, et al., 1968; Sulzbacher and Costello, 1970). On the other hand, it is virtually impossible to teach grammar without using morphology and phonology at the same time (Gray and Fygetakis, 1968 a and b; Fygetakis and Gray, 1970). Although we might define our program as a grammar program in order to define its emphasis, it should be realized that phonology and morphology are also involved.

Figure 5 Completed Schematic of the Instructional Equation for Language Training

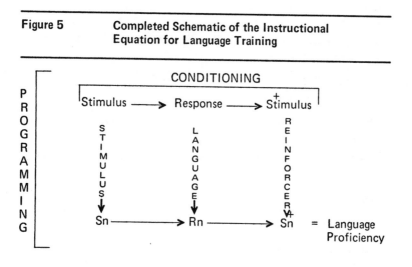

Summary

We mentioned earlier the futility of conditioning into the behavior all
language forms and all verbal responses. Our alternative is to develop a
conditioning system whereby the child gains the facility to spontaneously generate correct and appropriate constructions within a given
corpus.
    Within the structure of this mini-language, it could be
hypothesized that the child would be able to incorporate new words
and rules into the corpus without specific conditioning. This self
perpetuation concept is critical to the success of the procedure. If
programmed conditioning does not teach the rules of the language, only
stereotyped responding will result. On the other hand, if programmed
conditioning does teach the basic as well as surface structure performance, then language will develop.

References

Ayllon, T. and Azrin, N. *The token economy.* New York: Appleton-
    Century-Crofts, 1968.

Bandura, A. *Principles of behavior modification.* New York: Holt,
    Rinehart and Winston, 1969.

Berko, J. The child's learning of English morphology. *Word,* 1958, *14,*
    150-177.

Chomsky, N. *Aspects of the theory of syntax.* Cambridge: M.I.T. Press,
    1965.

Chomsky, N. Topics in the theory of generative grammar. In T. Sebeak
    (Ed.), *Current trends in linguistics,* Vol. III. The Hague: Mouton,
    1966.

Chomsky, N. The general properties of language. In F. Darley (Ed.),
    Brain mechanisms underlying speech and language. New York:
    Grune and Stratton, 1967a.

Chomsky, N. Review of Skinner's verbal behavior. In L. Jakobovits and M. Miron (Eds.), *Readings in the psychology of language.* Englewood Cliffs, N. J.: Prentice-Hall, 1967b.

Dixon, T. and Horton, D. (Eds.) *Verbal behavior and general behavior theory.* Englewood Cliffs, N.J.: Prentice-Hall, 1968.

Englemann, S. How to construct effective language programs for the poverty child. In F. Williams (Ed.) *Language and poverty.* Chicago: Markham, 1970.

Eysenck, H. *Behavior therapy and the neuroses.* London: Pergamon Press, 1960.

Fodor, J. and Katz, J. (Eds.) *The structure of language.* Englewood Cliffs, N. J.: Prentice-Hall, 1964.

Fygetakis, L. and Gray, B. Programmed conditioning of linguistic competence. *Behaviour Research and Therapy*, 1970, *8*, 153-163.

Gray, B. Behaviorism, linguistics, binary logic and information theory: Are Skinner and Chomsky really compatible? In D. Mowrer (Ed.), *Modification of speech behavior.* Tempe: Arizona State University, 1969.

Gray, B. Language acquisition through programmed conditioning. In R. Bradfield (Ed.), *Behavior modification: The human effort.* San Rafael: Dimensions Press, 1970.

Gray, B. and Fygetakis, L. Mediated language acquisition for dysphasic children. *Behaviour Research and Therapy,* 1968a, *6*, 263-280.

Gray, B. and Fygetakis, L. The development of language as a function of programmed conditioning. *Behaviour Research and Therapy,* 1968b, *6*, 455-460.

Guess, D. A functional analysis of receptive language and productive speech: Acquisition of the plural morpheme, *Journal of Applied Behavior Analysis,* 1969, *2*, 55-64.

Guess, D., Sailor, G., and Baer, D. An experimental analysis of linguistic development: The productive use of the plural morpheme. *Journal of Applied Behavior Analysis,* 1968, *1*, 297-306.

Hendershot, C. *A bibliography of program and presentation devices.* Saginaw: Scher Printing Co., 1964.

Jakobovits, L. and Miron, M. (Eds.) *Readings in the psychology of language.* Englewood Cliffs, N. J.: Prentice-Hall, 1967.

Krasner, L. and Ullmann, L. (Eds.). *Research in behavior modification.* New York: Holt, Rinehart and Winston, 1965.

Lee, L. Developmental sentence types: A method of comparing normal and deviant syntactic development. *Journal of Speech and Hearing Disabilities,* 1966, *31*, 311-330.

Lee, L. A screening test for syntax development. *Journal of Speech and Hearing Disabilities,* 1970, *35,* 103-112.

Lenneberg, E. The capacity for language acquisition. In J. Fodor and J. Katz (Eds.), *The structure of language.* Englewood Cliffs, N. J.: Prentice-Hall, 1964.

Lenneberg, E. On explaining language. *Science,* 1969, *164,* 635-643.

Lillywhite, H., Bradley, D., Nelson, D., Holeman, L., Nicon, J., and Fletcher, S. *Oregon Language Profile.* Personal communication, 1970.

Lovaas, I. A program for the establishment of speech in psychotic children. In H. Sloane and B. MacAulay (Eds.), *Operant procedures in remedial speech and language training.* Boston: Houghton Mifflin, 1968.

McCarthy, D. Language development in children. In L. Carmichael (Ed.), *Manual of child psychology,* 2nd ed. New York: John Wiley & Sons, 1954.

McNeill, D. Developmental psycholinguistics. In F. Smith and G. Miller (Eds.), *The genesis of language.* Cambridge: M.I.T. Press, 1966.

McNeill, D. On theories of language acquisition. In T. Dixon and D. Horton (Eds.), *Verbal behavior and general behavior.* Englewood Cliffs, N. J.: Prentice-Hall, 1968.

Menyuk, P. *Sentences children use.* Cambridge: M.I.T. Press, 1969.

Meyerson, L. Discussed in A behavioral strategy for reading training. B. Gray. In R. Bradfield (Ed.), *Behavior modification of learning disabilities*. San Rafael: Academic Therapy Publications, 1971.

Mykelbust, H. *Auditory disorders in children*. New York: Grune and Stratton, 1957.

Pipe, P. *Practical programming*. New York: Holt, Rinehart and Winston, 1966.

Skinner, B. *Verbal behavior*. New York: Appleton-Century-Crofts, 1957.

Skinner, B. Teaching machines. *Science,* 1958, *128*, 969-977.

Sloane, H. and MacAulay, B. (Eds.) *Operant procedures in remedial speech and language training*. Boston: Houghton Mifflin, 1968.

Smith, F. and Miller, G. *The genesis of language*. Cambridge: M.I.T. Press, 1966.

Sulzbacher, S. and Costello, J. A behavioral strategy for language training of a child with autistic behaviors. *Journal of Speech and Hearing Disorders,* 1970, *35*, 256-276.

Wolpe, J. *Psychotherapy by reciprocal inhibition*. Palo Alto: Stanford University Press, 1958.

Wyatt, G. *Language learning and communication disorders in children*. Toronto: The Free Press, 1969.

Yates, A. *Behavior therapy*. New York: John Wiley and Sons, 1970.

2 Programs

The purpose of this chapter is to show the application of the principles described in Chapter One to the development of language programs. The delivery system (programmed conditioning) and the content (language) are further defined and demonstrated through specific programs.

      The first part of this chapter will be devoted to discussion of the delivery system and the variables involved. The second part will present several sample language programs including placement and branching procedures. The third part of the chapter will concern the language content or the selection of grammatical forms to be taught.

The Delivery System

The delivery system is composed of a series of steps arranged in a logical sequence. Each step is derived from consideration of a number of important variables. In addition to the basic variables of stimulus, response, and consequence discussed in Chapter One, Gray and Fygetakis (1968) identified six other variables: model, reinforcement schedule, criterion, stimulus mode, response mode, and complexity. These nine variables are considered in the development of a program and program steps. Each of them will be discussed in some detail.

1. Response. This variable refers to the desired response by the child. It may be in two modalities: oral and nonoral. The oral response length may vary and is often a critical element in the oral language responses of children (Templin, 1957; Lee, 1966; Menyuk, 1964, 1969; Bloom, 1970; McNeill, 1966). The response must be clearly defined and described so that its presence or absence may be reliably detected. The success of any program is contingent upon the correct response evaluation. Commonly, programs start with short, easy responses which are gradually increased in length and complexity.

2. Stimulus. The stimulus refers to that class of events which precedes the response and sets the stage for its occurrence. The stimuli are commonly visual and/or auditory. They may take the form of objects, actions, pictures, or verbal utterances by the teacher. In language programs, pictures or verbal utterances by the teacher are used. The verbal utterance tells the child what grammatical form he is to learn to say. The picture gives him semantic information about the words used in the utterance.

3. Reinforcer. The reinforcer describes the consequence which is to be used. Commonly, tokens (styrofoam stars, chips, beans, etc.) are given to the child. These are later exchanged for toys. The child may select his own reinforcers from a list or group of them. He must earn enough tokens to "buy" or exchange them for an item. The reinforcer should be specified before the program starts. Another form of reinforcer is the utterance, "Good," which is said after every correct response. It is paired with and delivered simultaneously with the token reinforcer.

4. Criterion. This variable refers to the standard of performance of the child. It sets the limit of his behavior so that the teacher will know when to move him ahead in the program. A criterion of ten successively correct responses is the common criterion for each step, if the child is working in a group of three or more children. If the child is working alone or with one other child, the criterion is doubled to twenty. In some programs with a large number of different responses the common criterion may be raised to twenty also.

5. Reinforcement Schedule. The schedule of delivery of a reinforcer or token is important. Usually when teaching a new skill or bit of language behavior, the reinforcement schedule is high—a token for every correct response (100 percent reinforcement). As the child learns the skill, the amount of token reinforcement is faded out. First to every other correct response (50 percent), then to every tenth correct response (10 percent), and finally to no token reinforcement at all, but merely social or verbal reinforcement such as "Good." Throughout the program the social reinforcement is delivered on a 100 percent schedule for correct responses, only the token reinforcement is gradually faded.

6. Response Mode. The response mode is divided into oral and nonoral categories. These categories could be further divided into subcategories. Nonoral responses include pointing, writing, body gesture, etc. Since the program is an oral language program, the response mode is usually oral language.

7. Stimulus Mode. As described in the section on the stimulus, there are several forms of stimuli. The two modes most often used are visual and auditory. Both visual (picture, objects, action) and auditory (a verbal utterance) stimuli are presented in the language programs.

The stimulus and response modes are combined to show their interrelationships:

Stimulus Mode		Response Mode	
Visual	Auditory	Oral	Nonoral
————	————	Oral	————
Visual	————	Oral	————
————	Auditory	Oral	————
Visual	Auditory	Oral	————
————	Auditory	————	Nonoral
Visual	Auditory	————	Nonoral
Visual	————	————	Nonoral

It can be seen that the lowest level of behavior would require a nonoral response to a visual stimulus and the highest level of behavior would require an oral response to no obvious stimulus. This concept of sequencing in programming aids in designing the sequence to move from easy steps to more difficult ones.

8. Model. The model variable refers to a special kind of stimulus which helps the child know exactly what he is to say. In programming language, it is a prompt. Whereas the stimulus is the total final target of what the child will eventually be able to say spontaneously at the end of a program, the model is that part of the stimulus which the child is expected to produce at a given point in the program. The models themselves are gradually faded so that the child must "remember" what he is supposed to say with no prompting. The five models are shown below:

Models	Explanation
IC Immediate Complete	The child is given the entire model of what he is to say just before he is to say it.
DC Delayed Complete	The child is given the entire model but it must be "held" briefly before he says the response.

IT Immediate Truncated	The child is given only a portion of what he is to say in the model immediately before he says it.
DT Delayed Truncated	The child is given only a portion of what he is to say in the model, and it must be "held" briefly.
N No Model	The child is given no model of what he is to say.

The model, therefore, is introduced early in the program to tell the child what to say and then it is gradually faded out as the child becomes more proficient in generating his own sentences.

The relationship between the stimulus and model is:

Stimulus	Model
picture "The ball is red."	"is" (IC)
then,	
picture "The ball is red."	"ball is red" (IC)
then,	
picture "The ball is red."	"ball" (IT)

9. Complexity. This is the variable which describes the relationship between the model and the response. The number of units in the model is related to the number of units in the response. If the model is one unit long and the response is one unit long, the complexity is 1-1. If the model is four units long and the response is four units long, then the complexity is 4-4. If the model is one unit long and the response is four units long, the complexity is 1-4. The complexity variable aids the programmer in evaluating the difficulty of the step and/or sequence he has chosen. All of the nine variables, subclassifications of each, and examples are shown in Table 1.

Table 1   The Nine Variables in Programmed Conditioning, Subclasses of Each, and Examples of Steps

Stimuli	Models	Response	Schedule	Criterion	Reinforcers	Stimulus Mode	Response Mode	Complexity
Objects Actions Pictures Verbal	IC DC IT DT N	Varying in Length (1-8 words)	100 50 10	10 20	Tokens Social	Visual Auditory	Oral Nonoral	0-1 1-1 2-2 3-3 2-3 n-n
				Examples				
(Step 37) Object	DC	A sentence of 5 words	50	20	Tokens and Social	Visual	Oral	5-5
(Step 5) Picture Verbal	IT (first word)	A sentence of 3 words	10	10	Tokens and Social	Visual Auditory	Oral	1-3

When designing and constructing a program, the programmer starts with variable one (response) and works through all up to variable nine (complexity). When branching or altering a program, the programmer starts with variable nine (complexity) and works backwards in an effort to reduce the difficulty of the program and increase its efficiency. It is important to keep in mind the interrelationships of the variables.

Number of Steps

To give some idea of the program sequence which could be generated with these nine variables, consider only the first six and their possible interrelationships. The other three variables—response mode, stimulus mode, and complexity—are not included in this calculation because they do not actually represent steps per se. There are a number of options for the variables in each step:

Stimuli		Models		Response		Schedule		Criterion		Reinforcers		Total Steps
4	(X)	3-17*	(X)	1-8	(X)	3	(X)	2	(X)	2		= 3,840

Using only the first six variables and the alternatives available, it is possible to derive a program sequence of 3,840 steps to teach one language form eight units (words) long. This sequence would be awkward to put on paper and difficult to administer. It would probably result in overtraining and take a long time for a child to complete. In order to simplify the strategy, the number of options for most of the variables were reduced. The six variables and their reduced options are:

Stimuli	Models	Response	Schedule	Criterion	Reinforcers	Total Steps
Pictures	IC	Oral	100%	10/20	token/social	
and/or	DC		50%			
Verbal	IT		10%			
	DT					
	N					
1 (X)	3-17 (X)	1-8 (X)	3	(X) 1	(X) 1	= 240

---

* Truncation steps reflect response length (there are 1-7 truncation steps for each DT and IT model contingent upon response length).

This resulted in a program model which is based on only 240 steps. From these steps were selected an average five steps per sequence for actual use in the program. Such a sequence is called a series. Any given program is made up of several of these five-step series. The typical program contains seven series or a total of 35 steps. The breakdown from possible (3840) to usable (240) to selected (5) steps for a series is shown below.

Possible	Usable	Selected
1	1	1
768	48	2
1536	96	3
2304	144	4
3840	240	5

The usable steps are available for branching purposes. All of the 240 steps will be shown later in this chapter in the discussion of branching procedures.

Program Logic

The program logic which includes both the overall design, or sequence of the program, and the nine variables to be used is shown in Figure 6.

In the right hand portion of Figure 6 is the overall program sequence. SE-A is an abbreviation for Series A. If one follows the arrows straight down from SE-A to SE. . .N, it can be seen that the program proceeds from Series A to the Nth Series—Series N. This is essentially a linear program (Cram, 1961; Pipe, 1966). However, not all children will be able to move through the program without error. Hence, branching procedures or extra steps may be needed to help the child through Series A—Series N. These are shown by the various SE-A', SE-B', SE—C'. . .SE-N' series. Each program is constructed to run quickly, effectively from SE-A to SE-N, but additional procedures (branching) are available in the event that the child has difficulty with the main series. These branching series (SE-A'—SE-A'-N') always bring

Figure 6　　　　　Program Logic and Nine Variables

Variables	Sequence
1. Response (Response)	
2. Stimulus (Stimulus)	
3. Reinforcer (R+)	
4. Criterion (C)	
5. Reinforcement Schedule (Sch.)	
6. Response Mode (RM)	
7. Stimulus Mode (SM)	
8. Model (M)	
9. Complexity (Cx)	

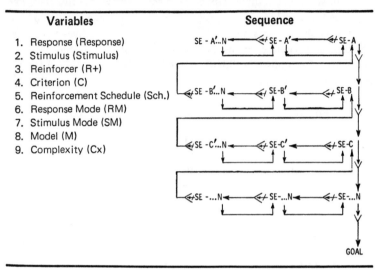

GOAL

the child back to the main series (SE-A—SE-N).

In the left hand portion of Figure 6 are shown the nine variables arranged in the order in which they are considered in the development of a program. Adjustments or branching processes are initiated by starting with variable nine and working back up through the sequence.

This scheme should be viewed as a philosophy of programming which is logical and systematic. It is to be used by the teacher and programmer to aid in the construction of any program for the teaching of any behavior. Some of the nine variables will receive more attention in the development of a program than in the branching processes. Different content will require different emphasis. This is only one program strategy. The reader should refer to Sloane and MacAulay (1968) and Girardeau and Spradlin (1970) for other forms.

Sample Programs: Construction and Execution

The logic system is used to select and arrange the variables into a programmed conditioning for language program consisting of series, steps, stimulus, model response, schedule of reinforcement, placement, and branching index. These will be shown in sample language programs

Table 2   Language Curriculum

A   Core

1 Identification of nouns
2 Naming nouns
3 In/on
4 Is
5 Is verbing
6 Is interrogative
7 What is
8 He/she/it
9 I am
10 Singular noun present tense
11 Plural nouns present tense
12 Cumulative plural/singular present tense
13 The

B Secondary

14 Plural nouns are
15 Are interrogative
16 What are
17 You/they/we
18 Cumulative pronouns
19 Cumulative is/are/am
20 Cumulative is/are/am interrogative
21 Cumulative what is/are/am

22 Cumulative noun/pronoun/ verb/verbing
23 Singular and plural past tense (t and d)

C Optional

24 Was/were
25 Was/were interrogative
26 What was/were
27 Does/do
28 Did
29 Do/does/did interrogative
30 What is/are doing
31 What do/does/did
32 Negatives not
33 Conjunction and
34 Infinitive to
35 Future tense to
36 Future tense will
37 Perfect tense has/have
38 Adjectives
39 Possessives
40 This/that/a
41 Articulation

with examples. The latter two (branching and placement) will be discussed more fully later. There are 41 programs including an articulation program. The entire curriculum is shown in Table 2. There is a separate program for each grammatical form to be taught.

Because of the length and similarity of the programs, only the "Is" (No. 4), and "Is" Interrogative (No. 6), and part of the "What Is" (No. 7), and an outline of the "Articulation" (No. 41) programs will be shown. These programs have been selected because they demonstrate the basic features of the programs and some important differences among them, especially between statement programs and question programs. The entire set of 41 programs is available elsewhere (Gray and Ryan, 1971). The programs are all constructed and executed in a similar manner.

The programs have been partially coded to reduce their length. In order to read the programs the code must be known. The code is shown in Table 3.

Table 3   The Code and Examples of Various Language Forms Used in the Programs

			Code		
Code	Decoded	Example	Code	Decoded	Example
N	= noun	"ball"	Ving	= verbing	"hitting"
Ns	= nouns	"balls"	Vtd	= verbed	"walked", "batted", "grabbed"
S	= subject	"boy"	Adv.	= adverb	"walked *fast*"
Ss	= subjects	"boys"	Adj.	= adjective	"the *blue* ball"
Pr	= pronoun	"he"	np	= noun phrase	"the ball'
/or//	= or, N/Ns	"ball" or "balls"	vp	= verb phrase	"is red"
P	= preposition	"in"	np-vp	= noun phrase-verb-phrase	"The ball is red."
V	= verb	"hit"			
Vs	= verbs	"hits"			

Sometimes the specific word is written out such as "the, and, in, does, is, was," etc. Use these specific words.

Decoded Statement Examples

Coded	Example
The S is N/Adj.	"The boy is captain/old" but use only "The boy is captain" or "The boy is old."
Is the S Ving?	"Is the dog barking?"
The S is Ving.	"The girl is walking."
Are the Ss P the N?	"Are the boys in the house?"
The S is Ving the N.	"The boy is walking the dog."
What is the S Ving?	"What is the girl holding?"
The Ss are Ving.	"The boys are jumping."
What are the Ss Ving?	"What are the boys kicking?"
The Ss V.	"The cats run."
The S Vs.	"The cat runs."
The S/Ss Vtd.	"The boy jumped" or "The boy jumped."
The S Vs N/Adv.	"The dog bites men" or "The dog bites hard."
The S is P the N.	"The car is in the garage."
Pr is P the N.	"He is in the car."

"Is" Program No. 4. The "Is" program (No. 4) is the first program in the sequence to require a sentence such as *"boy is old"* or *"boy is in house."* The "Is" program No. 4 in coded form is shown in Figure 7.

      Read the program from the top. The title is the "Is" program, the target is "S is N/Adj./PN" (Subject is Noun or Adjective or Preposition Noun). There will be no placement procedures used. The teacher will accept the use of "the" in the response as correct although

Figure 7   The "Is" Program No. 4 Coded

Target:	S is: N/Adj.//PN		Steps:	22		
Comments:	No Placement		R+:	Redeemable Tokens		
	Accept Addition of "the"		Criterion:	10/20		
	in the Response as Correct					

Step	Stimulus	Model	Response	Sch	P	BI
	Take criterion test					
	Start					
Series A						
1	Pictures np–vp (The S is N/Adj.)	IC	is	100		245
2	Pictures np–vp	IC	is N/Adj.	100		5
3	Pictures np–vp	IC	S is N/Adj.	100		17
4	Pictures np–vp	DC	S is N/Adj.	50		27
5	Pictures np–vp	IT (S)	S is N/Adj.	50		32
6	Pictures np–vp	DT (S)	S is N/Adj.	50		38
7	Pictures np–vp	N	S is N/Adj.	10		43
Series B						
1	Pictures np–vp (The S is P the N)	IC	is P	100		245
2	Pictures np–vp	IC	is P N	100		17
3	Pictures np–vp	IC	S is P N	100		35
4	Pictures np–vp	IT (S is P)	S is P N	50		49
5	Pictures np–vp	IT (S)	S is P N	50		56
6	Pictures np–vp	DT (S)	S is P N	50		63
7	Pictures np–vp	N	S is P N	10		70
Series C						
1	Pictures Combinations np–vp (The S is: N/Adj.//P the N)	IC	S is N/Adj.//PN	100		245
2	Pictures Combinations np–vp	IT(S)	S is N/Adj.//PN	50		29
3	Pictures Combinations np–vp	N	S is N/Adj.//PN	10		41

Figure 7, continued

Step	Stimulus	Model	Response	Sch	P	BI
Series D						
1	Pictures Questions (Is the S N/Adj.$_1$ or N/Adj.$_2$? What is N/Adj.? Is the S in the N$_1$ or the N$_2$? Where is the S?)	IC	S is N/Adj.//PN	100		245
2	Pictures Questions	IT (S)	S is N/Adj.//PN	50		29
3	Pictures Questions	N	S is N/Adj.//PN	10		41
Series E						
1	Story	N	S is N/Adj.//PN	10		245
Series F						
1	Conversation	N	S is N/Adj.//PN	10		245
	IHC					
	End of program Stop Take criterion test Go to next program					

it is not required. The "Is" program is program number four. There are 22 steps in the program. Redeemable tokens will be used along with social reinforcement. The criterion is ten or twenty successively correct responses for each step. The series and steps are listed in the first column. The series indicate a class of responses such as "S is N/Adj." (Subject is Noun or Adjective), and the steps indicate each step in the series. Each new series denotes a basic change in the response, e.g., Series B, "The S is P the N," etc.

The stimulus column indicates what will be used as stimulus events. The child first takes a Criterion Test (more about Criterion Testing in Chapter Three) and then is ready to start the program. The stimulus events are pictures and verbal np-vp (noun phrase-verb phrase, a sentence). The teacher makes up a sentence to go with the picture. The sentence must be "The S is N/Adj." ("The boy is captain" or "The boy is tall"). The model is indicated in the next column and in the first step it is IC (immediate complete). The response is "is" which is what the child is to say. The Sch (schedule) column tells about the schedule of reinforcement. In Step One it is 100 percent

Figure 8   An Illustration of a Language Program, Series A,
Step I, of the "Is" Program No. 4

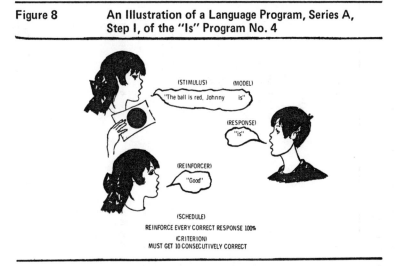

(STIMULUS)   (MODEL)
"The ball is red, Johnny   is"

(RESPONSE)
"is"

(REINFORCER)
"Good"

(SCHEDULE)
REINFORCE EVERY CORRECT RESPONSE 100%
(CRITERION)
MUST GET 10 CONSECUTIVELY CORRECT

or a token for each correct response. The P (placement) column comes
next, but there is no placement in the "Is" program (No. 4). Finally the
BI (branch index) indicates the steps to use if a child is failing a step.
An illustration of the language program in action is shown in Figure 8.

Read through the program noting the various models,
the gradual increase in length of response, the change in reinforcement
schedules, and the two different responses (Series A, "S is N/Adj." and
Series B, "S is PN"). All programs go through the basic series, move to
a combination series (Series C in the "Is" program), to a question
series (Series D), to a story series (Series E), and finally to a conversation series (Series F). The IHC at the end of the program indicates
Initiate Home Carryover (see Chapter Three). The Criterion Test is
taken again, and the child goes to the next program.

Note that the stimulus is changed from pictures and
verbal statements to pictures and questions and finally to only questions.
The sentences themselves are continually changed. The response is at
first very small, just the one word, "is." It gradually is expanded to
"Subject is noun," or "Adjective," or "Subject is preposition noun."
The article, "the," is not required but it is accepted as correct if the
child uses it. The reinforcement schedule starts high (100 percent) and
terminates low (10 percent). Keep in mind that the verbal reinforcer,
"Good," is given on a 100 percent schedule for correct responses.

In Figure 9 the same "Is" program (No. 4) with each
step decoded is presented. Because the criterion is always ten or twenty
and the P (Placement) and BI (Branch Index) are not of concern at this
time, they are not shown in the decoded program.

Figure 9   The "Is" Program No. 4 Decoded with Examples of Each Step

Step	Stimulus	Child's Name	Model	Response	Schedule
Series A					
1	Pictures np–vp (The S is N/Adj.)		IC	is	100
	The boy is old.	Johnny	Is	is	Give token for each correct response.
2	Pictures np–vp		IC	is N/Adj.	100
	The girl is young.	Johnny	is young	is young	Give token for each correct response.
3	Pictures np–vp		IC	S is N/Adj.	100
	The car is blue.	Johnny	Car is blue.	Car is blue.	Give token for each correct response.
4	Pictures np–vp		DC	S is N/Adj.	50
	The boy is happy.	Johnny		Boy is happy.	Give a token for every other correct response.
5	Pictures np–vp		IT(S)	S is N/Adj.	50
	The dog is brown.	Johnny	Dog	Dog is brown.	Give a token for every other correct response.
6	Pictures np–vp		DT(S)	S is N/Adj.	50
	The boy is captain.	boy, Johnny		Boy is captain.	Give a token for every other correct response.

32

No.	Stimulus	Prompt			Count	Reinforcement
7	Pictures / np–vp / The girl is sad.	Johnny	N	S is N/Adj. — Girl is sad.	10	Give token for every 10 correct responses.

Series B

No.	Stimulus	Prompt			Count	Reinforcement
1	Pictures / np–vp / (The S is P the N) / The boy is on the floor.	Johnny	IC — is on	is P — is on	100	Give token for each correct response.
2	Pictures / np–vp / The girl is in the house.	Johnny	IC — is in house	is P N — is in house	100	Give token for each correct response.
3	Pictures / np–vp / The dog is in the yard.	Johnny	IC — Dog is in yard.	S is P N — Dog is in yard.	100	Give token for each correct response.
4	Pictures / np–vp / The car is on the street.	Johnny	IT (S is P) — Car is on	S is P N — Car is on street.	50	Give token for every other correct response.
5	Pictures / np–vp / The man is on the wall.	Johnny	IT (S) — Man	S is P N — Man is on wall.	50	Give token for every other correct response.
6	Pictures / np–vp / The boy is in the car.	boy, Johnny	DT(S)	S is P N — Boy is in car.	50	Give token for every other correct response.

33

Figure 9, continued[*]

Step	Stimulus	Child's Name	Model	Response	Schedule
7	Pictures np–vp The girl is in the room.	Johnny	N	S is P N Girl in in room.	10 Give token for every 10 correct responses.
Series C					
1	Pictures Combinations np–vp (The S is N/Adj.// P the N) The boy is old. or The girl is on the grass.	Johnny	IC Boy is old. or Girl is on grass.	S is: N/Adj.// P N	100 Give token for each correct response.
2	Pictures Combinations np–vp The girl is pretty. or The dog is in the yard.	Johnny	IT(S) Girl or Dog	S is N/Adj.// P N Girl is pretty. or Dog is in yard.	50 Give token for every other correct response.
3	Pictures Combinations np–vp The man is old. or The dog is on the chair.	Johnny	N	S is N/Adj.// P N Man is old. or Dog is on chair.	10 Give token for every 10 correct responses.

Series D

1

Pictures

Questions

(Is the S N/Adj.$_1$ or N/Adj.$_2$?
What is N/Adj.?
What N/Adj. is the S?
Is the S in the N$_1$ or the N$_2$? Where is the S?)

Question		IC			
Is the boy old or young?	Johnny	Boy is old.	S is N/Adj.// P N	100	
or		or			
What is blue?	Johnny	Car is blue.	Boy is old.		Give token for each correct response.
or		or	or		
What color is the house?	Johnny	House is red.	Car is blue.		
or		or	or		
Is the girl in the house or the yard?	Johnny	Girl is in yard.	House is red.		
or		or	or		
Where is the dog?	Johnny	Dog is on chair.	Girl is in yard.		
			or		
			Dog is on chair.		

2

Pictures

Questions

Question		IT(S)			
Is the girl happy or sad?	Johnny	Girl	S is N/Adj.// P N	50	
or		or			
What is old?	Johnny	Man	Girl is happy.		Give token for every other correct response.
or		or	or		
What color is the dog?	Johnny	Dog	Man is old.		
or		or	or		
Is the boy on the grass or on the porch?	Johnny	Boy	Dog is white.		
or		or	or		
Where is the girl?	Johnny	Girl	Boy is on porch.		
			or		
			Girl is in yard.		

35

Figure 9, continued

Step	Stimulus	Child's Name	Model	Response	Schedule
3	Pictures Questions		N	S is N/Adj.// P N	10
	Is the lady pretty or ugly?	Johnny or		Lady is pretty. or	Give token for every 10 correct responses.
	What is blue?	Johnny or		House is blue. or	
	What color is the dress?	Johnny or		Dress is green. or	
	Is the man in the car or the house?	Johnny or		Man is in car. or	
	Where is the dog?	Johnny		Dog is on grass.	
Series E					
1	Story	Johnny	N	S is N/Adj.// P N	10
	Teacher tells a simple story using story book and asks questions as in the question series.			Boy is tired. or Snake is in tree.	Give token for every 10 correct responses.
Series F					
1	Conversation	Johnny	N	S is N/Adj.// P N	10
	Teacher engages in simple conversation using questions as in the question series			Boy is happy. or Bird is in tree.	Give token for every 10 correct responses

"Is Interrogative" Program No. 6. Most of the programs require the child to generate statements using various grammatical forms. A group of eleven programs also teach the child to ask questions. These programs are the same as the statement programs except for the question (command) series. In the "Is Interrogative" program (No. 6) the child is taught to ask an "is" question such as "Is dog in house?" The entire "Is Interrogative" program (No. 6) is shown in coded form in Figure 10.

The name of the program is the "Is Interrogative" program. The target is the grammatical forms: "Is S: N/Adj.? Ving? P N? Ving N/Adv? Ving P N?" ("Is subject noun" or "adjective? Is subject verbing? Is subject preposition noun? Is subject verbing preposition noun?"). The comments indicate that the teacher should accept, but not require, the use of the word "the" in the response. It is program number six. There are 35 steps in the program. Reedemable tokens are used reinforcers. The criterion is ten or twenty successively correct responses in each step before moving to the next step. The child takes a Criterion Test and is put through a placement process before starting the program. Read through the program noting the various grammatical forms, models, stimuli, responses, and schedules. There are five basic series which teach the new forms (Series A-E), a combination series (Series F) to combine the forms, a command series (Series G), a story series (Series H), and finally a conversion series (Series I). At the end of the program the IHC (Initiate Home Carryover) program is executed. The child takes a post program Criterion Test. If he passes it, he moves to the next program.

Figure 10   The "Is Interrogative" Program No. 6 Coded

Target:	Is S: N/Adj.? Ving? P N? Ving N/adv.? Ving P N?		Steps: R+:	35 Redeemable Tokens		
Comments:	Accept Addition of "the" in the Response as Correct		Criterion:	10/20		

Step	Stimulus	Model	Response	Sch	P	Bl
	Take criterion test Placement Start					
Series A						
1	Pictures Questions (Is the S N/Adj.?)	IC	Is	100	0	245
2	Pictures Questions	IC	Is S	100		5
3	Pictures Questions	IC	Is S N/Adj.?	100	1	17

Figure 10, continued

Step	Stimulus	Model	Response	Sch	P	BI
4	Pictures Questions	DC	Is S N/Adj.?	50		27
5	Pictures Questions	IT (Is)	Is S N/Adj.?	50	2	32
6	Pictures Questions	DT (Is)	Is S N/Adj.?	50		38
7	Pictures Questions	N	Is S N/Adj.?	10	3	43
Series B 1	Pictures Questions (Is the S Ving?)	IC	Is S Ving?	100		251
2	Pictures Questions	DC	Is S Ving?	50	4	27
3	Pictures Questions	IT (Is)	Is S Ving?	50		32
4	Pictures Questions	DT (Is)	Is S Ving?	50	5	38
5	Pictures Questions	N	Is S Ving?	10		43
Series C 1	Pictures Questions (Is the S P the N?)	IC	Is S P N?	100	6	251
2	Pictures Questions	IT (Is S P)	Is S P N?	50		49
3	Pictures Questions	IT (Is)	Is S P N?	50	7	56
4	Pictures Questions	DT (Is)	Is S P N?	50		63
5	Pictures Questions	N	Is S P N?	10		70
Series D 1	Pictures Questions (Is the S: Ving the N? Ving N/Adv.?)	IC	Is S Ving N/Adv.?	100	8	251
2	Pictures Questions	IT (Is S Ving)	Is S Ving N/Adv.?	50		49
3	Pictures Questions	IT (Is)	Is S Ving N/Adv.?	50	9	56
4	Pictures Questions	DT (Is)	Is S Ving N/Adv.?	50		63
5	Pictures Questions	N	Is S Ving N/Adv.?	10		70

Step	Stimulus	Model	Response	Sch	P	BI
Series E						
1	Pictures Questions (Is the S Ving P the N?)	IC IT	Is S Ving P N?	100	10	252
2	Pictures Questions	(Is S Ving P)	Is S Ving P N?	50		76
3	Pictures Questions	IT (Is)	Is S Ving P N?	50	11	84
4	Pictures Questions	DT (Is)	Is S Ving P N?	50		95
5	Pictures Questions	N	Is S Ving P N?	10	12	103
Series F						
1	Pictures Combinations Questions (Is the S: N/Adj.? Ving? P the N? Ving the N? Ving N/Adv.? Ving P N?)	IC	Is S: N/Adj.? Ving? P N? Ving N/Adv.? Ving P N?	100		247
2	Pictures Combinations Questions	IT (Is)	Is S: N/Adj.? Ving? P N? Ving N/Adv.? Ving P N?	50	13	29
3	Pictures Combinations Questions	N	Is S: N/Adj.? Ving? P N? Ving N/Adv.? Ving P N?	10		41
Series G						
1	Pictures Commands (Show picture *after* child asks a question.) I see a S, guess if the S is: N/Adj.$_1$ or N/Adj.$_2$! P the N$_1$ or P the N$_2$! Ving$_1$ or Ving$_2$! Ving the N$_1$ or the N$_2$! Ving P the N$_1$ or P the N$_2$! Ving N/Adv.$_1$ or N/Adv.$_2$!)	IC	Is S: N/Adj.? Ving? P N? Ving N/Adv.? Ving P N?	100	14	245

Figure 10, continued

Step	Stimulus	Model	Response	Sch	P	BI
2	Pictures Commands	IT (Is)	Is S: N/Adj.? Ving? P N? Ving N/Adv.? Ving P N?	50		29
3	Pictures Commands	N	Is S: N/Adj.? Ving? P N? Ving N/Adv.? Ving P N?	10	15	41
Series H 1	Story	N	Is S: N/Adj.? Ving? P N? Ving N? Ving P N?	10		245
Series I 1	Conversation	N	Is S: N/Adj.? Ving? P N? Ving N? Ving P N?	10	16	245

IHC

End of Program
Stop
Take criterion test
Go to next program

Only Series A and Series G of the "Is Interrogative" program (No. 6) are shown decoded in Figure 11 because the other series are similar in format to the "Is" program (No. 4).

"What Is" Program No. 7. In addition to the interrogative programs there are also programs which teach "Wh" question forms such as "What is." The basic procedures are the same except for the series (Series G) where the child is commanded to ask a "Wh" question. The "command" series is the same as the "question" series of the statement programs. Series G of the "What is" program (No. 7) is shown below in Figure 12.

Figure 11   Series A and G of the "Is Interrogative" Program No. 6 Decoded with Examples of Each Step

Step	Stimulus	Child's Name	Model	Response	Schedule
Series A					
1	Pictures		IC	is	100
	Questions				
	(Is the S N/Adj.?)				
	Is the boy happy?	Johnny	is	is	Give token for each correct response.
2	Pictures		IC	is S	100
	Questions				
	Is the dog brown?	Johnny	is dog	is dog	Give token for each correct response.
3	Pictures		IC	Is S N/Adj.?	100
	Questions				
	Is the man old?	Johnny	Is man old?	Is man old?	Give token for each correct response.
4	Pictures		DC	Is S N/Adj.?	50
	Questions				
	Is the girl young?	Johnny		Is girl young?	Give token for every other correct response.
	Is girl young?				
5	Pictures		IT (is)	Is S N/Adj.?	50
	Questions				
	Is the lady pretty?	Johnny	Is	Is lady pretty?	Give token for every other correct response.
6	Pictures		DT (Is)	Is S N/Adj.?	50
	Questions				
	Is the cat hungry?	Johnny	Is	Is cat hungry?	Give token for every other correct response.

41

Figure 11, continued

Step	Stimulus	Child's Name	Model	Response	Schedule
7	Pictures Questions Is the book black?	Johnny	N	Is S N/Adj.? Is book black?	10 Give token for every 10 correct responses.
Series G 1	Pictures Commands Show picture *after* child asks question. I see a S. Guess if the S is: N/Adj.$_1$ or N/Adj.$_2$! P the N$_1$ or P the N$_2$! Ving$_1$ or Ving$_2$! Ving the N$_1$ or the N$_2$! Ving P the N$_1$ or P the N$_2$! Ving N/Adv$_1$ or N/Adv$_2$!		IC	Is S: N/Adj.? Ving? P N? Ving N/Adv.? Ving P N?	100
	I see a boy. Guess if the boy is: happy or sad! or	Johnny	Is boy happy? or	Is boy happy? or	Give a token for each correct response.
	in the house or in the yard! or	Johnny	Is boy in yard? or	Is boy in yard? or	
	running or walking! or	Johnny	Is boy walking? or	Is boy walking? or	

	kicking the ball or the house! or	Johnny	Is boy kicking ball? or	
	running in the street or in the yard! or	Johnny	Is boy running in street? or	
	walking fast or slow!	Johnny	Is boy walking fast?	
2	Pictures Commands	IT (is)	Is S: N/Adj.? Ving? P N? Ving N/Adv.? Ving P N?	50
	I see a girl, Guess if the girl is:			Give token for every other correct response.
	young or old! or	Johnny or	Is	Is girl young? or
	sitting or standing! or	Johnny or	Is	Is girl standing? or
	in the car or in the house! or	Johnny or	Is	Is girl in car? or
	holding the book or the ball! or	Johnny or	Is	Is girl holding book? or
	jumping in the yard or in the street! or	Johnny or	Is	Is girl jumping in street? or
	laughing loudly or softly!	Johnny	Is	Is girl laughing softly?
3	Pictures Commands	N	Is S: N/Adj.? Ving? P N? Ving N/Adv.? Ving P N?	10

Figure 11, continued

Step	Stimulus	Child's Name	Model	Response	Schedule
	I see a man, Guess if the man is:				Give a token for every 10 correct responses.
	tall or short!	Johnny		Is man tall?	
	or	or		or	
	laughing or talking!	Johnny		Is man talking?	
	or	or		or	
	on the floor or on the table!	Johnny		Is man on table?	
	or	or		or	
	swinging the baby or the cat!	Johnny		Is man swinging cat?	
	or	or		or	
	walking on the roof or on the floor!	Johnny		Is man walking on floor?	
	or	or		or	
	kicking hard or softly!	Johnny		Is man kicking hard?	

Figure 12   Series G (Commands) of the "What Is" Program No. 7 Decoded with Examples of Each Step

Step	Stimulus	Child's Name	Model	Response	Schedule
Series G 1	Pictures Command (Show picture *after* child asks question.) I see something. N/Adj. Ask me what! I see something Ving Ask me what! Something is P the N. Ask me what! I see the S Ving something. Ask me what! Something is Ving P the N. Ask me what! I see something green. Ask me what! or I see something running. Ask me what! or Something is in the house. Ask me what! or		IC	What is N/Adj.? Ving? P N? S Ving? Ving? P N?	100
		Johnny or		What is green? or	Give a token for each correct response.
		Johnny or		What is running? or	
		Johnny or		What is in the house? or	

45

Figure 12, continued

Step	Stimulus	Child's Name	Model	Response	Schedule
	I see the man kicking something. Ask me what!	Johnny		What is the man kicking?	
	or			or	
	Something is walking on the table. Ask me what!	Johnny		What is walking on the table?	
2	Pictures Commands		IT (What)	What is: N/Adj.? Ving? P N? S Ving? Ving P N?	50
	I see something old. Ask me what!	Johnny	What	What is old?	Give token for every other correct response.
	or	or		or	
	Something is on the floor. Ask me what!	Johnny	What	What is on floor?	
	or	or		or	
	I see something walking. Ask me what!	Johnny	What	What is walking?	
	or	or		or	
	Something is running on the street. Ask me what!	Johnny	What	What is running on the street?	

3	Pictures Commands	N	What is: N/Adj.? Ving? P N? S Ving? Ving P N?	10	Give a token for every 10 correct responses.
	I see something happy. Ask me what!	Johnny	What is happy?		
	or	or	or		
	I see something playing. Ask me what!	Johnny	What is playing?		
	or	or	or		
	Something is in the yard. Ask me what!	Johnny	What is in yard?		
	or	or	or		
	The boy is throwing something. Ask me what!	Johnny	What is boy throwing?		
	or	or	or		
	Something is in the house. Ask me what!	Johnny	What is in the house?		

"Articulation" Program No. 41. The articulation program is not a formal part of the language programs but is an important ancillary program. Experience has shown that children's articulation improves as a result of the language training process; however, a number of children may start the language training process with severe articulation problems. In addition, some of the programs require special phonemes as semantic markers such as /s/ or /z/ in the plurals and present tense programs. Certain consonant clusters will occur which include both the semantic marker (/s/ or /z/) and another consonant (/tʃ/ or /ʃ/) such as /ʃəz/ in words like "bushes" or "watches." These are difficult and children may make errors as a result of the semantic marker /s/ or /z/ being in a consonant cluster. A child might be able to produce the final /s/ sound in "house" but be unable to produce the /s/ when in combination with other consonants, such as /ts/ in "cats" or /gz/ in "dogs."

The articulation program is especially designed to teach children the articulation of these special consonant sounds in certain phonetic combinations. The articulation program is written in the same format as the language programs and is administered the same way. Any sound may be taught in the format. Because of this, a presentation of the entire articulation program in this chapter would be somewhat redundant. Only the series outline is shown in Table 4. You will note that the program runs in the same sequence as most common articulation therapy procedures (Van Riper, 1963; Johnson, et al.,1965).

Table 4	Outline of Series in Articulation Program No. 41 Steps: 38 (7 optional)

Series	Target
A	sound in isolation
B	sound in nonsense syllable in initial position
C	sound in nonsense syllable in final position
D	sound in blend nonsense syllable (optional)*
E	sound in words initial, medial, final position
F	sound in one of two words
G	sound in sentence
H	sound in sentence in response to questions
I	sound in sentence in story (optional)*
J	sound in sentence in conversation (optional)*

*Optional series take into consideration the age of the child, the language level of the child, and the fact that the child is constantly exposed to the sounds at the conversational and story level in language programs and show and tell time.

The sounds morphemically critical for the language program are /s/ and /z/. Less critical are /t/ and /d/. Contingent upon an evaluation of the child's articulation, the teacher may decide that a given child does not need articulation training on these sounds. In that event, the teacher may either institute articulation training on other sounds or have no articulation training program at all.

We recommend that only a small part (five percent) of the time for therapy be devoted to articulation training if the decision is made that the child needs it. This training should begin at the same time as the first language program with one of the above-mentioned sounds. Hence the child will be working through language programs for 95 percent of his therapy time and through an articulation program five percent of his time. If he starts on one of the first language programs, he may get to the sentence level in the articulation program before he is capable of generating a sentence. In that case, he is moved on to the next sound at the beginning series of the program.

It is seldom necessary to utilize the story and conversation series because so much of this level of speech is already going in the language programs themselves. When a child reaches this level (story and conversation), his articulation performance in the language program can be monitored.

The blend series is optional because many young, preschool children have great difficulty with consonant blends. This becomes somewhat critical in the plural and present tense programs where the child must add the phonetic marker /s/ or /z/ to nouns and/or verbs. He may have difficulty in combinations such as / z/ in a word like "wishes." A simple resolution to this problem is to permit articulatory deviation of the blend but to hold the child to producing some approximation of the /s/ or /z/ marker, such as /wɪʔɪz/. Repeated stimulation with the correct articulation provided by the language programs usually takes care of this articulatory deviation. If the teacher believes this not to be the case with an individual child, additional articulation training may be instituted using the same articulation program on these special, difficult consonant clusters.

The focus of the language programs is correct grammatic production which approximates appropriate articulation. The high density of stimulation built into the program usually provides for the acquisition of normal articulation. It would be an error to spend a disproportionate amount of time in articulation training when the child's basic problem is grammar, and improvement in that area is often "spontaneously" accompanied by improvement in articulation.

Stimulus Pictures and Sentences

The "Is" (No. 4) program, and selected series of the "Is Interrogative" (No. 6) program, "What is" (No. 7) program, and an outline of the "Articulation" (No. 41) program have been shown. The same basic procedures are used throughout the rest of the 37 programs. The teacher must be able to read (decode) the programs, look at a picture, and generate an appropriate stimulus sentence. A desired sentence form is always written out enclosed in parentheses marks in the first step in each series. These same grammatical forms (coded) will be used over and over again throughout the program.

Any type of pictures may be used. They should be chosen to portray a wide variety of people, places, activities, numbers, and things. Advertising photographs cut out of contemporary magazines are especially clear and colorful. These may be pasted to construction paper to aid in manipulation and durability. The teacher may want to divide the pictures into subcategories of (1) plurals, (2) singulars, and (3) male-female. Commonly, all of the pictures will be appropriate for most programs. The teacher can make up a grammatical stimulus sentence regardless of the picture, but it should be as semantically accurate as possible. The sentence should match the correct number, sex, color, etc. of the pictures.

The teacher should attempt to have as much content variety as possible in the stimulus sentences. A strength of the program lies in the wide variety of sentences generated by the teacher. In a real sense, the teacher is demonstrating the kind of language behavior the child is to learn. It is important that the teacher have normal articulation and language.

Models

The five models have been shown in the preceding programs. The model is a prompt to the child about the response the teacher wants him to make. In the first steps in a program or series the child is given complete models. It also may be helpful to exaggerate the target form in the first few steps in a series. In the final steps the child is given no model. The model is determined by the response. The teacher needs to know both the model form (IC—immediate complete, for example) and the response ("S is N/Adj.," for example) to generate the right model. The model information tells the teacher how much of the response should be given in the model. The response tells the teacher the exact response desired from the child so that the model may be made to fit the response. The five models with examples of each are reviewed in Table 5.

Table 5

Table 5   **The Five Models, Three Basic Sequences, and Examples**

The models are:

IC	Immediate Complete	All the response
DC	Delayed Complete	All the response delayed
IT	Immediate Truncated	Part of the response
DT	Delayed Truncated	Part of the response delayed
N	None	None

The three basic sequences are:

1	Stimulus	Child's Name	Model (IC, IT)	Child's Response
2	Stimulus	Model (DC, DT)	Child's Name	Child's Response
				Child's Response
3	Stimulus	None (N)	Child's Name	

The examples are:

Stimulus	Model	Child's Name	Model	Response
"The S is N/Adj"		Johnny	IC "is"	"is"
"The S is N/Adj"		Johnny	IC "is N/Adj"	"is N/Adj"
"The S is N/Adj"		Johnny	IC "S is N/Adj"	"S is N/Adi"
"The S is N/Adj"	DC "S is N/Adj"	Johnny		"S is N/Adj"
"The S is N/Adj"		Johnny	IT ("S") "S"	"S is N/Adj"
"The S is N/Adj"	DT ("S") "S"	Johnny		"S is N/Adj"
"The S is N/Adj"	(N)	Johnny		"S is N/Adj"

     In each truncated model, the specific grammatical parts to be presented are shown in parentheses. For examples, IT (S) = Immediate Truncated. The teacher just says "S", e.g., "Boy."

Response Evaluation

After the child has responded, the teacher must immediately decide whether or not his response was correct. In general the child must give the response listed in the response column, but there are exceptions. The response evaluation, rules, and examples are shown below.

Error	Response	Child's Response	Evaluation
1. Misarticulated	Is	"Id"	(correct)
2. The wrong word but the correct grammar	Is big	"Is small"	(correct)
3. Child says too much	Is	"Is big"	(incorrect)
4. Child says too little	Is big	"Is"	(incorrect)

5. Unintelligible	Is big	"Cdxdjt"	(incorrect but not scored)
6. No response	Is big	"_____"	(incorrect but scored only as NR or no response)
7. Two tries	Is big	"Are big, is big"	(incorrect)

It will be noted in the examples that the child is permitted great variation in both articulation and semantics. The goal of the program is correct grammar, hence initially the child is rewarded for correct, recognizable grammar although the actual words uttered may be misarticulated or not semantically appropriate. Experience has shown that after several programs the children gradually become both phonetically and semantically accurate. If a child should persist in giving semantically inaccurate words after several programs, this standard should be tightened and he should be reinforced for only correct semantic reproductions. Should articulatory deviation persist, the child's age and his progress on the articulation program should be taken into consideration.

Occasionally children will "jump" ahead in a program. They will give a response for Step 3 when they are supposed to give a response for Step 1. Although the child is right in the sense that this response will be eventually desired and reinforced, his response is evaluated as incorrect. The reason for this is that some children will begin guessing about what is desired of them which may result in a high frequency of inaccurate guessing. It is better to keep the child under the control of the program.

Another point concerns the difference between evaluation and scoring. Evaluation refers to the decision about the accuracy of the response. Scoring is the process of recording this information. Commonly, responses evaluated as correct or incorrect are scored and recorded accordingly. However, in examples five and six, the evaluation of the response is that it is incorrect but the scoring is different. An "unintelligible response" is incorrect, but it is not scored. A "no response" is also incorrect, but it is scored only as NR (no response) rather than as right or wrong. Scoring will be discussed in more detail in Chapter Three. Special consideration must be made for the word, "the." The stimulus presentation always contains the word, "the." The models and responses for the first twelve programs do not. Experience has indicated that the addition of even one word, such as "the," tends to overload the young or severely language handicapped child as he is learning basic grammar. In a sentence such as "The boy is in the house," or "The boy is kicking the ball," two "the's" increase the grammatic-syntactic load by 33 percent and this combination is especially difficult. For older children or children with language ability acquired on the early programs, the use of the word, "the," is not such a problem. The programs solve this problem by permitting the child to use "the," if he is capable; and/or picks it up from the stimulus presentations, but not holding him responsible for "the" until program (No. 13) which teaches "the."

Another special case is contractions such as "isn't" and "he's." Contractions in the program are scored wrong. Children will normally use contractions outside the program; but when working in a program, they must demonstrate both units so that the teacher will be sure the children know them.

Reinforcement

After a child has made a response, the evaluation is made immediately. If it was correct, the teacher is to say "Good" and give him a token immediately. The teacher is to say nothing and move on to the next stimulus presentation if the child is incorrect. For example:

Response	Child's Response	Reinforcement
Is	"Is"	"Good" and give token.
Is	"Are"	Nothing, go on to next item.

The child is always told "Good" when he is right, but he is given tokens only on a special schedule which is listed in the program script. For example:

Schedule	Reinforcement
100 = 100 percent	Give a token for each correct answer.
50 = 50 percent	Give a token for every two correct answers or for every other correct answer.
10 = 10 percent	Give a token for every ten correct answers or for every tenth correct answer.

This information is illustrated in the following:

<u>100% schedule</u>

Teacher: "The ball is red, Johnny, is."

Johnny: "Is."

Teacher: "Good." (Gives token also.)

<u>50% Schedule</u>

Teacher: "The ball is red, Johnny, the ball is red."

Johnny: "Ball is red."

Teacher: "Good." (Does not give token, but gives token only for every other correct response.)

<u>10% Schedule</u>

Teacher: "The ball is red, Johnny."

Johnny: "Ball is red."

Teacher: "Good." (Does not give token, but gives token only for every tenth correct response.)

<u>Incorrect Response</u>

Teacher: "The ball is red, Johnny."

Johnny: "Ball red."

Teacher: (Nothing, goes on to next item.)

The reinforcement schedule of 100 percent is a fixed ratio schedule, i.e., one reinforcer for each correct response. The reinforcement schedule of 50 percent is also a fixed ratio schedule, i.e., one reinforcer for every two correct responses or every other correct response; however, in actual practice teachers often vary this schedule so that they are still giving a reinforcer 50 percent of the time. But they may let more than two correct responses go without reinforcement and reinforce each of the next few correct responses; this results in a variable ratio reinforcement schedule with a mean 50 percent base. The same is true of the 10 percent schedule. It is important to fade the schedule (100 percent to 50 percent to 10 percent), but it is often difficult for the teacher to do it perfectly. Therefore, some variation around the mean of 50 percent or 10 percent is acceptable and perhaps even desirable. Variable ratio reinforcement schedules are very powerful in maintaining behavior (Ferster and Skinner, 1956).

Series Sequence

The series in each program is designed to start the child with the new form to be taught, e.g., "is, is verbing, the," etc. Within the first series, the child is taken through an increase in response length until he is using the new form in sentences. At this point in the series, the models and reinforcement schedules are gradually faded until at the end of each series the child is producing the sentence with no model and only 10 percent token reinforcement'

Each subsequent series teaches the new form with a different verbal complement ("N/Adv., P N, N/Adj."). After all the desired verbal complements have been taught singularly, they are combined in a combination series where they are all presented randomly, interchangeably.

After the combination series, comes the question or command series. In this the child must use all of the combined forms in response to questions or commands with minimal information given him by the teacher through models.

Next comes the story series where the stimulus is composed of a simple story from a story book told by the teacher. The teacher then asks questions, makes comments, etc. to evoke all the forms taught previously in the program. For beginning children, the stories are kept simple and within the child's verbal repertoire. As the students progress, the stories can become more complex.

Finally, comes the conversation series during which the teacher uses only natural stimuli and questions to evoke the desired forms. Initially, conversation is simple—at the level of the child's language ability. Later the conversation can be more normal and more complex.

Placement

At the top of the next to last column on each program script is a symbol, "P." This stands for placement. Placement refers to the process of placing a child within a program. Most children will start a program at the beginning and work all the way through each step. Occasionally older children who have some language or those who have been through several programs will be able to start in a program at a step beyond the first one. Placement is administered after the Criterion Test and just before the child starts a program. The placement system shown in Figure 13 will aid in determining just where a child should begin. By dividing each program into sixteen fairly equal divisions, the placement process permits the teacher to place a child in a program by sampling only four program steps. The placement system is used from the "Is verbing" program through the rest of the programs with the exception of the cumulative programs.

Figure 13   **The Placement Process and Table of Placement Numbers**

1. Using the table below and the placement (P) numbers in the program script go through the various program steps.
2. For each step the child must score two out of three attempts successively correct to pass.

   Pass   Pass   Fail   and   Fail   Pass   Pass   =   Pass

3. Continue to test until a P item, 15P for example, is reached. This is the point of entry into the program and the child should begin the program at this step.

Table of Placement Numbers

Test	Pass	Fail
8	12	4
12	14	10
14	15	13
15	16	14P
4	6	2
6	7	5
7	7P	6P
2	3	1
1	1P	0P
10	11	9
9	9P	8P
13	13P	12P
11	11P	10P
3	3P	2P
5	5P	4P
16	--	15P

The placement test process consists of three presentations of the program step designated by the placement number. The child must score two successively correct responses to earn a pass on that step. If he responds correctly to presentations one and two, or to presentations two and three, he will score pass. Anything other than this is counted as a failure. An example of the placement procedure is shown below:

	Placement	Program Step	Response
1.	8	Series D, Step 1	child fails
2.	4	Series B, Step 2	child passes
3.	6	Series C, Step 1	child fails
4.	5	Series B, Step 4	child passes
5.	Child starts program at 5P or Series B, Step 4		

The teacher starts testing the child with Placement 8 (actually, the corresponding program step) and continues to test steps as indicated by the child's pass or fail performance. The teacher should administer the step similar to regular programming with the exception that no token or verbal reinforcement is given. The corresponding program step to Placement 8 on the "Is Interrogative" (No. 6) Program is Series D, Step 1, "Is the S Ving N/Adj? " If the child fails that step he goes to Placement 4. He is then tested on the corresponding program step. If he passes Placement 4, he is then tested on Placement 6. If he fails 6, he is then tested on Placement 5. If he passes 5, he starts the program on 5. The starting step is Series B, Step 4. The P behind the number as in 5P, 14P, 8P, 4P, etc. indicates where to start the program.

By using the placement system the teacher can "locate" the child within a program very quickly. However, we recommend no placement for the first three programs (no. 1, no. 2, no. 3) because occasionally the placement process will place a child too high. This is especially true of non-English speaking and echolalic children. It will become clear in the first few program steps that the child is placed too high because the child will demonstrate excessive difficulty with the step (below 50 percent accuracy or ten consecutive errors in the first session). If the teacher suspects the child is placed too high, the entire placement procedure should be readministered. If the child places lower on the second test, then he should be started at the new placement step. If the child places again as high or higher, then he should be moved back to the first step in the preceding series. This should be continued, if necessary, until the child's performance in the program indicates that he is placed properly.

Branching

Branching is the process whereby the teacher uses additional instructions and/or steps to help a child who is having difficulty on a particular program step. Only a few branching procedures will be necessary for most children in most programs. Commonly, children will make some errors in initial programs as they go through the process of learning the protocol for the various models, especially the response to IT and DT models. Errors will occur in the first step in each new series as the child learns the new form to be taught. Some children will demonstrate behavior problems which increase errors on the program. This usually signifies that they need behavior control rather than language branching procedures. The programs are designed to run at an average 90 percent accuracy which means there will be error responses. Hence, it is important that the teacher not overreact to error. The teacher must know when to branch and what procedures to use. The criteria for when to branch and three specific branch procedures will be discussed below.

Instructions. The first type of branching activity is additional verbal instructions to go along with the step. The instruction is presented immediately before the model. This procedure is instituted when a child demonstrates ten consecutive error responses of the same kind. In a combination, question or command, story and conversation series this means ten consecutive errors on one or more of the forms. The instructions are given no more than three times. If they are going to be effective, this will be shown in the first few attempts. It is important that they not become either "crutches" or reinforcement for the child's error.

A variation of instruction is to simply emphasize the target word or error response as part of the model. Two examples are:

"The ball is red, Johnny, Ball *IS* red."

"The balls are red, Johnny, Ball*S* are red."

This type of instruction should be used first in response to any number of different kinds or errors. If this fails, another forms of instruction should be used.

The choice of instruction is often indicated by the type of error. Common errors and their corresponding instructions are shown below.

Error	Instruction
Child's response is too short	"Say the whole thing" or "Say what I say."
Child's response is too long	"Say only what I say."
Child's first response is wrong, but he corrects himself	"Say it right the first time."
Child omits important word in response	"Remember to say _____ (the key word)."
Child omits final /s,z/ marker	"We say _____/s,z/ (exaggerage /s,z/)."

An example of the placement of an instruction would be:

Stimulus	Instruction	Model
"The ball is red,	(say the whole thing)	Johnny, ball is red."

Often instructions alone will improve a child's performance. If the instructions do not help the child and he demonstrates ten more consecutive errors, go to the Branch Index (BI) (the second type of branching). If the instructions improve the child's performance but he continues to perform under 80 percent correct for three sessions, move to the basic Branch Index (BI).

Basic Branch Index. The Branch Index (BI), is composed of 240 steps using the common variation in models, response length, and reinforcement schedules. The BI is put into use when a child demonstrates ten consecutive errors after instructions (twenty total) or when the child demonstrates performance which is under 80 percent accuracy for three sessions. The entire Branch Index with the 240 steps is shown in Figure 14. The steps are carried out in the same manner as the regular program steps.

Figure 14   The Branch Index

C = Continue in the program. Return to the program step.

Criterion: is 10 in all steps except for special steps in certain programs. When child is working in one-to-one or two-one situations, the criterion is doubled or 20.

The subscript in the IT and DT models ($_1$) tells the number of words to put in the model. DT_2 means put in the first two words of the response.

Branch Index	Model	Response Length	Schedule	Pass	Fail
1	IC	1	100	C	245
2	IC	1	50	3	245
3	IC	1	10	4	2
4	DC	1	100	5	3
5	DC	1	50	C	3
6	DC	1	10	7	245
7	N	1	100	8	6
8	N	1	50	9	7
9	N	1	10	C	7
10	IC	2	100	C	245
11	IC	2	50	12	245
12	IC	2	50	13	11
13	DC	2	100	14	12
14	DC	2	50	C	12
15	DC	2	10	16	245
16	IT_1	2	100	17	15
17	IT_1	2	50	C	15

Figure 14, continued

Branch Index	Model	Response Length	Schedule	Pass	Fail
18	IT_1	2	10	19	245
19	DT_1	2	100	20	18
20	DT_1	2	50	C	18
21	DT_1	2	10	22	245
22	N	2	100	23	21
23	N	2	50	24	22
24	N	2	10	C	22
25	IC	3	100	C	245
26	IC	3	50	27	245
27	IC	3	10	28	26
28	DC	3	100	29	27
29	DC	3	50	C	27
30	DC	3	10	31	245
31	IT_2	3	100	32	30
32	IT_2	3	50	33	31
33	IT_2	3	10	34	32
34	IT_1	3	100	35	33
35	IT_1	3	50	C	32
36	IT_1	3	10	37	245
37	DT_2	3	100	38	36
38	DT_2	3	50	39	37
39	DT_2	3	10	40	38
40	DT_1	3	100	41	39
41	DT_1	3	50	C	38
42	DT_1	3	10	43	245
43	N	3	100	44	42
44	N	3	50	45	43
45	N	3	10	C	43
46	IC	4	100	C	245
47	IC	4	50	48	245
48	IC	4	10	49	47
49	DC	4	100	51	48
50	DC	4	50	51	49
51	DC	4	10	52	50
52	IT_3	4	100	53	51
53	IT_3	4	50	C	49
54	IT_3	4	10	55	245
55	IT_3	4	100	56	54
56	IT_2	4	50	57	55
57	IT_2	4	10	58	56
58	IT_1	4	100	59	57
59	IT_1	4	50	C	56
60	IT_1	4	10	61	245
61	DT_3	4	100	62	60
62	DT_3	4	50	63	61

Branch Index	Model	Response Length	Schedule	Pass	Fail
63	DT_3	4	10	65	62
64	DT_2	4	100	65	63
65	DT_2	4	50	66	64
66	DT_2	4	10	67	65
67	DT_1	4	100	68	66
68	DT_1	4	50	C	63
69	DT_1	4	10	70	245
70	N	4	100	71	69
71	N	4	50	72	70
72	N	4	10	C	70
73	IC	5	100	C	245
74	IC	5	50	75	245
75	IC	5	10	76	74
76	DC	5	100	78	75
77	DC	5	50	78	76
78	DC	5	10	79	77
79	IT_4	5	100	80	78
80	IT_4	5	50	C	76
81	IT_4	5	10	82	245
82	IT_3	5	100	83	81
83	IT_3	5	50	84	82
84	IT_3	5	10	86	82
85	IT_2	5	100	86	84
86	IT_2	5	50	87	85
87	IT_2	5	10	88	86
88	IT_1	5	100	89	87
89	IT_1	5	50	C	84
90	IT_1	5	10	91	245
91	DT_4	5	100	92	90
92	DT_4	5	50	93	91
93	DT_4	5	10	94	92
94	DT_3	5	100	95	93
95	DT_3	5	50	98	92
96	DT_3	5	10	97	95
97	DT_2	5	100	98	96
98	DT_2	5	50	99	97
99	DT_2	5	10	100	98
100	DT_1	5	100	101	99
101	DT_1	5	50	C	95
102	DT_1	5	10	103	245
103	N	5	100	104	102
104	N	5	50	105	103
105	N	5	10	C	103
106	IC	6	100	C	245
107	IC	6	50	108	245
108	IC	6	10	109	107
109	DC	6	100	110	108
110	DC	6	50	111	109
111	DC	6	10	113	109

Figure 14, continued

Branch Index	Model	Response Length	Schedule	Pass	Fail
112	IT_5	6	100	113	111
113	IT_5	6	50	114	112
114	IT_5	6	10	115	113
115	IT_4	6	100	116	114
116	IT_4	6	50	C	111
117	IT_4	6	10	118	245
118	IT_3	6	100	119	117
119	IT_3	6	50	120	118
120	IT_3	6	10	122	118
121	IT_2	6	100	122	120
122	IT_2	6	50	123	121
123	IT_2	6	10	124	122
124	IT_1	6	100	125	123
125	IT_1	6	50	C	120
126	IT_1	6	10	127	245
127	DT_5	6	100	128	126
128	DT_5	6	50	130	127
129	DT_5	6	10	130	128
130	DT_4	6	100	131	129
131	DT_4	6	50	132	130
132	DT_4	6	10	136	128
133	DT_3	6	100	134	132
134	DT_3	6	50	135	133
135	DT_3	6	10	136	134
136	DT_2	6	100	138	134
137	DT_2	6	50	138	136
138	DT_2	6	10	139	137
139	DT_1	6	100	140	138
140	DT_1	6	50	C	132
141	DT_1	6	10	142	245
142	N	6	100	143	141
143	N	6	50	144	142
144	N	6	10	C	142
145	IC	7	100	C	245
146	IC	7	50	147	245
147	IC	7	10	148	146
148	DC	7	100	149	147
149	DC	7	50	150	148
150	DC	7	10	152	148
151	IT_6	7	100	152	150
152	IT_6	7	50	153	151
153	IT_6	7	10	154	152
154	IT_5	7	100	155	153
155	IT_5	7	50	C	150
156	IT_5	7	10	157	245
157	IT_4	7	100	158	156
158	IT_4	7	50	159	157
159	IT_4	7	10	160	158
160	IT_3	7	100	161	159
161	IT_3	7	50	164	158
162	IT_3	7	10	163	161

Branch Index	Model	Response Length	Schedule	Pass	Fail
163	IT_2	7	100	164	162
164	IT_2	7	50	165	163
165	IT_2	7	10	166	164
166	IT_1	7	100	167	165
167	IT_1	7	50	C	161
168	IT_1	7	10	169	245
169	DT_6	7	100	170	168
170	DT_6	7	50	171	169
171	DT_6	7	10	173	169
172	DT_5	7	100	173	171
173	DT_5	7	50	173	172
174	DT_5	7	10	174	173
175	DT_4	7	100	175	174
176	DT_4	7	50	180	171
177	DT_4	7	10	178	176
178	DT_3	7	100	179	177
179	DT_3	7	50	180	178
180	DT_3	7	10	182	178
181	DT_2	7	100	182	180
182	DT_2	7	50	183	181
183	DT_2	7	10	184	182
184	DT_1	7	100	185	183
185	DT_1	7	50	C	176
186	DT_1	7	10	187	245
187	N	7	100	188	186
188	N	7	50	184	187
189	N	7	10	C	187
190	IC	8	100	C	245
191	IC	8	50	192	245
192	IC	8	10	193	191
193	DC	8	100	194	192
194	DC	8	50	195	193
195	DC	8	10	196	194
196	IT_7	8	100	199	193
197	IT_7	8	50	198	196
198	IT_7	8	10	199	197
199	IT_6	8	100	201	198
200	IT_6	8	50	201	199
201	IT_6	8	10	202	200
202	IT_5	8	100	203	201
203	IT_5	8	50	C	196
204	IT_5	8	10	205	245
205	IT_4	8	100	206	204
206	IT_4	8	50	207	205
207	IT_4	8	10	208	206
208	IT_3	8	100	209	207
209	IT_3	8	50	212	206
210	IT_3	8	10	211	209
211	IT_2	8	100	212	210
212	IT_2	8	50	213	211
213	IT_2	8	10	214	212
214	IT_1	8	100	215	213
215	IT_1	8	50	C	209

Branch Index	Model	Response Length	Schedule	Pass	Fail
216	IT_1	8	10	217	245
217	DT_7	8	100	218	216
218	DT_7	8	50	219	217
219	DT_7	8	10	220	218
220	DT_6	8	100	222	218
221	DT_6	8	50	222	220
222	DT_6	8	10	223	221
223	DT_5	8	100	224	222
224	DT_5	8	50	225	223
225	DT_5	8	10	230	220
226	DT_4	8	100	227	225
227	DT_4	8	50	228	226
228	DT_4	8	10	229	227
229	DT_3	8	100	230	228
230	DT_3	8	50	233	227
231	DT_3	8	10	232	230
232	DT_2	8	100	233	231
233	DT_2	8	50	234	231
234	DT_2	8	10	235	233
235	DT_1	8	100	236	234
236	DT_1	8	50	C	225
237	DT_1	8	10	238	245
238	N	8	100	239	237
239	N	8	50	240	238
240	N	8	10	C	238

The Branch Index (BI) starts with one word responses and increases to eight word responses. All of the different models including different truncations and the three different schedules of reinforcement (100 percent, 50 percent, and 10 percent) are included in these steps.

The steps in each program have been selected from these 240 steps. The steps enclosed in double lines ("＝＝＝") are the program steps. Series A, Step 1, in the "Is" program is the same as BI, Step 1, in the Branch Index. Each step in the program script has a BI number which refers the teacher to the appropriate BI step.

When a child has been under 80 percent accuracy for three sessions, the teacher should note the BI number, refer to the BI steps, and institute the branch step. It will require the same response in most instances with only the model and/or reinforcement schedule changed, but the teacher should check the response length to be sure, the criterion will be either ten or twenty.

When working in the BI, the teacher uses different fail criteria. If the child demonstrates five consecutive errors, the teacher goes to the BI number listed in the fail column. If the child performs at under 80 percent accuracy for only one session, this is considered as a fail and the teacher moves the child back to the next BI number.

For example, in the "Is" (No. 4) program, Series B, Step 4, has a BI of 49. The teacher would then turn to the BI steps and find number 49. The BI number 49 is a DC model with 100 percent reinforcement. The response is the same. The teacher continues using the BI steps (51, 52, etc.), if the child passes them, until the child reaches a double-lined step ===(in this case, 53) with a C indicated in the pass column. This will be the step in the program which the child was failing. If he now passes this BI step, he returns to the program and repeats the program step. If the child continues to fail (48, 47, 46), he will eventually end up on BI 245, a special branch step which will be discussed later. This procedure is illustrated below:

Child fails Step 4, Series B, in "Is" (No. 4) Program (3 sessions under 80 percent, or 20 consecutive errors)

1. BI number is 49.
2. Go to BI step and find number 49 in left hand column.
3. 49 is a DC model.   100 percent   If pass, go to 52; if fail, go to 48.
4. 51 is a DC model.   10 percent   If pass, go to 52; if fail, go to 50.
5. 52 is an IT_3 model.   100 percent   If pass, go to 53; if fail, go to 51.
6. 53 is an IT_3 model.   50 percent   If pass, go back to program step Series B, Step 4; if fail, go to 49.

Special Branch Index Steps. In addition to the basic branch steps (1-240), there are some special branch steps (245-257). These will be discussed in some detail and examples given of each. The fail criteria are the same as for the basic Branch Index.

1. 245. This is a special procedure not found anywhere else in the Branch Index. This can mean that the step is too difficult and that additional preprogram or extraprogram activities are necessary. Commonly, this step refers to removing the stimulus pictures and/or np-vp and presenting only the model to the child. This could be a super model of "boy"-boy, "is"-is, "red"-red, or presenting the model one word at a time. Any procedure to help the child master the troublesome form is acceptable. Failure after 245 procedures would suggest abandoning the series, the program, or reevaluating the reinforcers.

2. 246. This is a truncation of the word to a sound or sounds. When a child is having consistent trouble moving from a Delayed Truncated (DT) model to No Model (N), it may be helpful to truncate the word to a sound. For example, DT ("Is") becomes 246 DT ("I"), or /ɪ/.

3. 247. This is a procedure used in the combination series only. The forms in the combination are broken down into pairs and each of these is taught, then combined, taught, combined, etc. The procedure is shown below:

Failure At	Pairs			
3 forms	1 + 2	2 + 3	1 + 3	
4 forms	1 + 2	3 + 4	1 + 2 + 3	2 + 3 + 4
5 forms	1 + 2	3 + 4	1 + 2 + 3	3 + 4 + 5
	1 + 2 + 3 + 4	and	2 + 3 + 4 + 5	

Example:

A child is in the "Is Verbing" (No. 5) program, Series D, Step 1 which combines "S is Ving, S is Ving N/Adv.," and "S is Ving P N" (three different forms). If the child is under 80 percent for three days, go to BI which is 247. Present these steps in the following way:

Step 247a "S is Ving" and "S is Ving N/Adv."

then

Step 247b "S is Ving N/ Adv." and "S is Ving P N"

then

Step 247c "S is Ving" and "S is Ving P N"

If child is successful, go back to Series D, Step 1 which combines all three forms.

Occasionally a child will have trouble with only one of the three forms. In that event select out the one troublesome form ("S is Ving PN", for example) and put the child through a step with only that form (IC model and 100 percent reinforcement schedule). When he passes the criterion (ten or twenty successively correct responses), put him back on the original program step: Series D, Step I.

4. 250-257. This is a procedure where the response length is decreased to the last word or words. Following the chart below, the response length is increased until the original length is reached (backward chaining). This series can also be used for forward chaining by starting with the first word or words and working through the 250-257 chart. All of these are done with an IC model and 100 percent reinforcement. The 250-257 chart follows:

No.	Response Length	Pass	Fail
250	1	251	245
251	2	252	250
252	3	253	251
253	4	254	251
254	5	255	252
255	6	256	252
256	7	257	253
257	8	C	253

Example:

A child is failing (three sessions under 80 percent) on the "Is Verbing" (No. 5) program, Series B, Step I, "S is Ving N/Adv." The BI is 251 on the 250-257 series. It indicates a response of two words but chained backwards, hence the step would be:

Step 251	IC Model	100 percent	Ving N/Adv.	If pass, go to 252; if fail, go to 250.
Step 252	IC Model	100 percent	is Ving N/Adv.	If pass, go to original program step; if fail, go back to 251.
Step 250	IC Model	100 percent	N/Adv.	If pass, go to 251; if fail, go to 245.

5. Combination, Question, and Command Series. Most of the series in the programs are written with five steps (the steps noted in double lines═══ in the BI). The combination, question, and command series are written with only three steps. The BI will take the child back to the second or fourth step not originally in the series. If he is successful, go to the next double-lined step in the BI (this is an exception to the rule about returning to the program step when a C is reached in the BI). If he successfully passes the second double-lined step, return to the program step according to the C. In other words, when the BI number refers to a double-lined step, the first time a C is encountered in the Pass column go to the next double-lined step in the BI. The second time a C is encountered return to the program step.

Example:

A child is failing (three sessions under 80 percent) in the "Is" (No. 4) program, Series D, Step 2. The BI is 29. In the Branch Index, BI 29 is a DC model at 50 percent reinforcement. Administer this step. If the child passes, go to the next double-lined step in the BI, Step 35, which is an IT_1 model at 50 percent reinforcement. If the child passes, return to the program step, Series D, Step 2. If the child fails, continue in the BI.

In the combination, question, and command series the BI responds to the response of the shortest length. When "S is N/Adj." and "S is P N" are being taught, the BI reflects "S is N/Adj." Therefore, many possible models are overlooked. The teacher can either work only on the defective form, "S is P N" for example, or present different models for the different responses. This is complicated, but it can be done.

6. Building a Response. In the first few series of some programs a response is built up from one word to a sentence in a very few steps. This procedure skips the basic BI steps that lie in between. The BI for these steps will take the child back to the middle step and if he is successful ($\overline{C}$), will put him back on the program. If he then fails the original program step again, the teacher must go back to the Branch Index itself and locate the intervening steps. It is important to check the response length in the BI.

Example:

A child fails (three days under 80 percent) for the "Is" (No. 4) program, Series A, Step 3, "S is N/Adj." The BI is 17 which takes the child back to "Is N/Adj.," IC Model, at 50 percent reinforcement. If the child passes this step, he is to continue, (C), in the program, i.e., go to the program step, Series A, Step 3. He could fail this step again and the teacher would have to go to the BI itself to find steps between. They would be 20, 24, all the intervening steps, and BI 17.

7. Reverberations. Reverberation means going up and down the same branch steps in a cycle, e.g., 143-144-143-144, etc. Two complete cycles or reverberations indicate that the teacher should start another branching procedure, perhaps a 245.

The fail criterion is the same in the special BI as in the basic BI steps. However, when working in a 245—which is the bottom level of the special BI steps—the teacher may continue in this step for a limited number of sessions, perhaps ten. At this point, serious consideration must be given to several alternatives. One alternative is to leave the series and go to another series; another alternative is to leave the program and go to another program which may be easier. A third is to develop an entirely new program which will prepare the child for the language program. A final choice is to dismiss the child as not being able to profit from the program and/or its branch procedures. This happens rarely, but on occasion it is the only reasonable procedure.

A summary of the various branch procedures and criteria for using them is shown in Figure 15.

Figure 15   An Outline of the Branching Procedures in Binary Logic

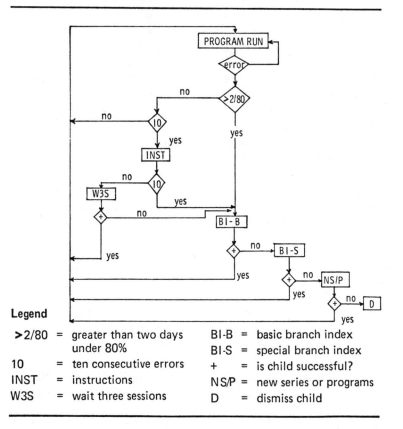

Legend

>2/80	=	greater than two days under 80%	BI-B	=	basic branch index
10	=	ten consecutive errors	BI-S	=	special branch index
INST	=	instructions	+	=	is child successful?
W3S	=	wait three sessions	NS/P	=	new series or programs
			D	=	dismiss child

The information is shown in binary logic form. In this figure the squares indicate operations and the diamonds indicate decisions. This analysis is based on answering the decision question either "yes" or "no."

The lines entering the diamonds on top and leaving them on the bottom are "yes" lines; lines leaving from either side are "no" lines. In the diamonds are questions which can be answered "yes" or "no"; in the squares are operations to be carried out depending upon the answers to the questions.

Starting at the top and working down we see first of all that we answer "yes" to the question that there is error in the program run. The next question, "Is the error greater than two days under 80 percent (> 2/80)," may be answered "yes" which indicates that we would go to the Branch Index (BI-B). If the answer was "no," we would then ask whether or not there were ten consecutive errors. If the answer was "no," we would continue on the program. If the answer is "yes," we would institute instructions (INST). After instructions we ask again, "Are there ten consecutive errors? If "no," we wait for three sessions (W3S). If "yes," we go to the Branch Index (BI-B). After waiting three days (W3S), we ask if the child was successful (+). If the answer is "no" (three days under 80 percent), we go to the Branch Index (BI-B). If the answer is "yes," we continue on the program. After the branching process (BI-B), we ask again if the child was successful (+). If "yes," we continue on the program; if "no," we go to the next special Branch Index (BI-S). After this branching process, we ask again if the child was successful (+). If the answer is "yes," we go on with the program. If the answer is "no," we go to alternative procedures such as new series or programs (N S/P). After these procedures are completed, we ask again if the child was successful (+). If the answer is "yes," we continue in the program. If the answer is "no," we dismiss the child. All the decisions and operations necessary in the branching process can be handled this way.

The branching process with instructions, basic branch index, and special branch procedures are available to the teacher if the child shows failure (ten or twenty consecutive errors or three sessions under 80 percent). The BI process (operating with five consecutive errors or one session under 80 percent) attempts to avoid overreaction to minimal error while providing immediate, powerful reaction to gross error.

Language Content

Programmed Conditioning for Language is a procedure for teaching spoken, oral language to nonusers. The emphasis is on oral language responses. There are three components of language: semantic, phonetic, and grammatic. There are also several modalities through which language may be perceived and expressed. These include speaking, hearing, writing, reading, gesturing, seeing, and so on. The emphasis in these programs is on spoken and heard language. This leaves decisions about semantic, phonetic, and grammatic aspects of oral language. Language teaching should include all of these elements, but the task appears overwhelming. One of the basic rules of behaviorism and/or programming is to start with specific behaviors and small steps; another is to select target behaviors which will be most helpful and meaningful to the learner. The resolution in this book has been to focus on the one element, grammar; however, grammar cannot be taught in isolation. Grammar is composed of words with meanings (semantic), and the words in turn are composed of sounds (phonetic). Hence, by focusing on grammar all three aspects of language are taught simultaneously. Grammar refers to a basic set of rules which permits the user to generate sentences. The verbalization of the rule is not required, but only the performance of language which indicates that the rule is known by the child.

Recent work in the past decade or so by linguists such as Chomsky (1957, 1965, 1969), Berko (1958), Bloom (1970), Brown and Fraser (1964), Klima and Belugi (1966), Lee (1966), Lee and Canter (1971), McNeill (1966), and Menyuk (1969) has opened new areas for the study of grammar in language. Their work has been described as transformational grammar or generative grammar. They have studied the language corpus and given us new systems for analyzing language. They have postulated new grammatical rules for the development of language. It is this focus upon the role of grammar in language development which has provided impetus for the content of the programs in this book. Not all the rules are clearly defined at this point in time and much work has yet to be done. There is enough, however, to help the language teacher and the language programmer to begin. The programmer's task is two-fold: he must select those grammatical forms which are most important and he must teach them in an appropriate sequence.

Selection of Forms

Ideally, the selection of forms should include: (1) a cross section of the various basic forms necessary to speak the language, (2) common forms

Table 6	List of Grammatical Forms with Examples Used in the Programs

	Form	Example
1	Nouns	Boy
2	Indefinite Pronouns	That
3	Personal Pronouns	I
4	Main Verbs	Is
5	Secondary Verbs	Want *to see*
6	Negatives	Not
7	Conjunctions	And
8	Interrogative Reversals	Is it red?
9	WH—Questions	What is it?
10	Prepositions	In
11	Adjectives	Blue
12	Possessives	His
13	Adverbs	Fast

which occur at high frequency, and (3) basic forms which the learner may use as building blocks or first steps to aid him in learning the more subtle, esoteric forms. For a cross section we went to the work of the linguists cited previously. The result is the cross section shown in Table 6 which includes many of the basic classes of grammatical structure.

In order to determine frequency of occurrence we went to the work of Berger (1968) which contained samples of conversational, spoken English. Most of the language forms taught in the programs have a relatively high frequency of occurrence. However, we had to extrapolate a great deal from Berger's data because there is little information on the frequency of occurrence of specific grammatical forms. Much research is needed in this area.

To select the appropriate basic forms was much more difficult since all of the fundamental forms have not yet been determined. Our compromise was to select forms which have some face validity in that they can be used to develop quite complex sentences and lead to several other forms of sentences. This state of affairs is shown in Figure 16. If a noun is taught, then a verb, and both are combined, we have a nucleus sentence composed of a subject and a verb. Both of these forms can then be expanded into noun phrases (np) and verb phrases (vp) respectively. Next, these same structures can be used in the question form. When pronouns, negatives, adjectives, adverbs, prepositions, possessives, and conjunctions are added into the basic np-vp paradigm

Figure 16

Figure 16   **A Tree Diagram Listing the Various Language Forms in the Language Programs and Their Possible Combinations**

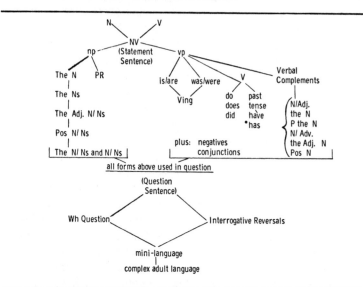

many complex sentences can be generated from these simple forms. The language forms chosen for these programs have the validity of giving the child many different grammatical classes of words and sequences which he can use to formulate a variety of new sentences. These forms appear to be enough to give the child a mini-language and the accompanying rules for learning more complex forms.

Sequence of Forms

It is important to teach the forms in an appropriate sequence. One choice is to follow the developmental data on the emergence of language forms presented in the work of the linguists cited previously. There is a strong inclination for the clinician to replicate the natural course of events. Another choice is to arbitrarily pick a sequence; still another is to teach the forms at random. Our choice was to put the forms in a sequence which appeared to have teaching value. When a child has

learned form $_1$, the next logical form is one which combines form $_1$ with another form, form $_2$, and so on until we have "chained" together all the forms which seem to fit with each other. Although this does not always follow the "natural" sequence of learning, it does appear to be a sound approach in programming technology. The programmer starts with behaviors which are already in the child's repertoire or need to be there in order for the child to learn more complex behaviors. This is somewhat arbitrary, program technology approach to developing a teaching sequence is best illustrated by examining the entire curriculum of the 41 programs as shown in Table 2 on page 27.

It can be seen in Table 2 that the first program is "Identification of Nouns" (No. 1). This is the only program in which the child's response is nonverbal. Next comes the "Naming Nouns" (No. 2) program in which the child is taught to say single nouns. The third program is the "In/On" (No. 3) program. This is a good illustration of programming strategy. Although prepositions do not normally occur in language immediately after a child has learned to say single nouns, they are important in this sequence because the child will need the prepositions for the rest of the programs from the "Is" (No. 4) program throughout. We teach "in" and "on" first and use them exclusively for several programs. In later programs (No. 8 and above), the teacher may use also "by" and "to" or rerun the "In/On" (No. 3) program with "by" and "to." Program No. 4 (Is) teaches the first sentences, "Subject is N/Adj." and "Subject is P N." Program No. 5 (Is Verbing) introduces both "verbing" and "adverbs." This program includes "Is Verbing," "Is Verbing N/Adv.," and "Is Verbing P N." It is logical in the program sense to go from "Is" to "Is Verbing" without the intermediate step of teaching "Verbs." Program No. 6 (Is Interrogative) and Program No. 7 (What Is) introduce the question forms of "Is" and "Is Verbing." Again, not the natural sequence but a logical next program to follow is "Is" and "Is Verbing." In Program No. 8, (He/She/It), the child is taught these pronouns to go with "Is" and "Is Verbing" along with the previous verbal complements of "N/Adj., N/Adv., and P N." Program No. 9, (I Am), teaches this common, useful pronoun and it is a logical extension of pronouns. It is used with "Is" and "Verbing" and the same verbal complements.

In Program No. 10, (Singular Noun Present Tense) the child is taught "S Verbs" (boy runs) all with regular verbs. We don't teach irregular verbs at this point because they are extremely difficult to teach and their frequency of occurrence, except for some special forms such as "do, does, did", is relatively low. We teach "S Verbs" (boy runs) before we teach "Ss Verb" (boys run) in Program No. 11 (Plural Nouns Present Tense) because we found that children learned them better in this sequence. We had no logic to help us in this choice, so we used the children's performance to guide us. Program No. 12, (Cumulative Plural/Singular Present Tense), is the first cumulative program where several different new forms (in this instance only two) are presented together. Program No. 13 (The) is the next program. We tried to teach "the" in earlier programs, but we found that it presented too much of a grammatic/syntactic overload. By Program No. 13 (The), the children have developed quite good language and are able to handle "the." Many of them will already be using it in their speech, and Program No. 13 (The) is in the curriculum at this point only to insure the fact that they do have it. From Program No. 13 (The) on, all the programs require the use of "the." Programs No. 1-13 comprise the "core" curriculum. Most of the children we have worked with have needed one or more of these programs. Once they have completed the "core" they often go through the other programs quite quickly and many even generalize or transform the forms from the first 13 programs and don't need many of the remaining programs.

Programs No. 14-16 teach "are," first with plural nouns and then in the two question forms: "are interrogative" and "what are." Program No. 17 presents "you, they, we." Programs No. 18-22 are cumulative programs which do not teach new forms, but merely review previously taught forms in conjunction with each other. These programs are of help in teaching contrasting forms such as "Boy is" and "Boys are." Program No. 23, (Singular and Plural Past Tense) teaches the basic past tense forms. Programs No. 14-23 constitute the secondary group of programs. Programs No. 14-17 and No. 23 are especially useful.

The optional group is composed of programs which teach "Was/Were" (No. 24-26), "Do/Does/Did" (No. 27-31), "Negatives" (No. 32), "Conjunction and" (No. 33), "Infinitive to" (No. 34), "Future tense to" (No. 35), "Future tense will" (No. 30), "Perfect tense has/have" (No. 37), "Adjectives" (No. 38), "Possessives" (No. 39), "This, That, A" (No. 40), and finally the "Articulation" program (No. 41). The sequence in the optional group is not as clear as in either the core or the secondary groups because these programs represent the cross section of forms to which most of the children generalize. The optional group may be viewed as a number of programs to teach necessary forms but not in any particular sequence.

The above comprises the present curriculum of the language programs. Most children will not need all of these programs. The responses vary in length from two to eight words. Hence, if different words are put into each category in each form, the actual number of "new" sentences which the child can generate after completing the program is very large. Table 7 illustrates this concept.

The number of steps in the programs varies. The early programs have fewer steps. The later programs average around 35 steps

Table 7   Programs, Forms, and Combined Forms

Programs (40)	Forms (55)
No. 2 Naming Nouns	*Nouns*
No. 4 Is	The subject *Is* Prep. the Noun
No. 15 Are Interrogative	*Are* the Subjects *Verbing?*
No. 27 Does/Do	The Subject *Does* Verb.
	The Subject *Do* Verb.
No. 39 Possessives	The Subject *Has* the Noun.

Combined Forms (158)
The Subject is Verbing Prep. the Noun

per program. This is because the five verbal complements, "N, the N, Adj., Adv., P the N" in combination with the other forms are used over and over again. The programs commonly have one basic five-step series to teach the new form and four five-step series to teach the new forms with the various verbal complements. In addition, there is one three-step series to combine forms, one three-step series for questions or commands, and two one-step series for story and conversation. Not all the verbal complements are taught in all the programs.

A basic form is something like "noun," "he," or "is interrogative." Besides the basic forms readily apparent in the titles of the various programs, there are comparative and superlative adjectives in the "Adjectives" (No. 38) program and possessives like "boy's, his," and "our" in the "Possessive" (No. 39) program. A combined form is a form in which two or more of the basic forms are used together such as "The subject is verbing the noun." The combination sentence is composed of six basic forms with one of the forms, "the," used twice.

Writing New Programs

The programs do not include all the various grammatical forms. Reflexive pronouns, passives, gerunds, irregular verbs, and past perfect, to mention a few, are not in the programs. If the teacher discovers that the child has not generalized from the mini-language to these additional forms, the teacher may want to write additional programs to teach them. Program writing using the language program format is not difficult. The teacher may follow the format used in the present programs including all of the nine variables. The teacher could refer to the BI for the steps, models, reinforcement schedules, etc. See Figure 17 for an outline form for writing new programs.

Suppose the teacher wanted to teach the passive form, "The subject is verbed by the noun" ("The girl is helped by the boy").

A child who has been through the programs knows the individual parts of this utterance; "The subject (The girl) is (is) verbed (helped) by the noun (by the boy)," but he has not yet combined the "is" with "verbed." Series A would teach this form by starting with Step 1, "is verbed," and ending with Step 7, "The subject is verbed." Series B

Figure 17   A Program Work Sheet

PROGRAM WORK SHEET
▲▲▲ monterey language program

NAME_____
PROGRAM_____
PROGRAM STEP_____
DATE_____

STEP	STIMULUS	MODEL	RESPONSE	SCH.	C	PASS	FAIL

FORM 104   DISTRIBUTED BY MONTEREY LEARNING SYSTEMS, INC. • 99 VIA ROBLES, MONTEREY, CALIFORNIA • ©1971, BEHAVIORAL SCIENCES INSTITUTE

would teach the entire statement, "The subject is verbed by the noun." There would be no need for a combination series. Only the question, story, and conversation series would follow; however, because the child would have substantial language at this time, the following forms could also be included: "The subject/subjects was/were verbed by the noun." If this were done, a combination series would be necessary.

The programs are open-ended. Any number of other grammatical forms can be taught in the same format. The important question is how many are needed until the child demonstrates adequate grammatical language.

Summary

This chapter has been concerned with the delivery system and the language content of the programs. Included were several sample programs and a description of how to run them. The language programs may appear to be extremely complex to teach on first examination. However, once the teacher learns the code and has some experience with the programs, they become relatively easy to administer.

References

Berger, K. The most common words used in conversations. *Journal of Communication Disorders,* 1968, *1,* 201-214.

Berko, J. The child's learning of English morphology. *Word*, 1958, *14,* 150-177.

Bloom, L. *Language development: Form and function in emerging grammars.* Cambridge: M.I.T. Press, 1970.

Brown, R. and Fraser, C. The acquisition of syntax. *Child Development Monographs*, 1964, *29,* 43-79.

Chomsky, C. *The acquisition of syntax in children from 5 to 10.* Cambridge: M.I.T. Press, 1969.

Chomsky, N. *Syntactic structures.* The Hague: Mouton, 1957.

Chomsky, N. *Aspects of the theory of syntax.* Cambridge: M.I.T. Press, 1965.

Cram, D. *Explaining teaching machines and programming.* San Francisco: Fearon Publishers, 1961.

Ferster, C. and Skinner, B. *Schedules of reinforcement.* New York: Appleton-Century-Crofts, 1956.

Girardeau, F. and Spradlin, J. (Eds.) A functional analysis approach to speech and language. 1970, *ASHA Monographs,* no. 14.

Gray, B. and Fygetakis, L. Mediated language acquisition for dysphasic children. *Behaviour Research and Therapy,* 1968, *6,* 263-280.

Gray, B. and Ryan, B. *Programmed conditioning for language: Program book.* Monterey, Calif.: Monterey Learning Systems, 1971.

Johnson, W., Brown, S., Curtis, J., Edney, C., and Keaster, J. *Speech handicapped school children,* rev. ed. New York: Harper and Bros., 1965.

Klima, E. and Belugi, W. Syntactic regularities in the speech of children. In J. Lyons and R. Wales (Eds.), *Psycholinguistic papers.* Edinburgh: Edinburgh University Press, 1966.

Lee, L. Developmental sentence types: A method for comparing normal and deviant syntactic development. *Journal of Speech and Hearing Disorders,* 1966, *31,* 311-330.

Lee, L. and Canter, S. Developmental sentence scoring: A method for measuring syntactic development in children's spontaneous *Journal of Speech and Hearing Disorders,* 1971, *36,* 315-340.

McNeill, D. Developmental psycholinguistics. In F. Smith and G. Miller (Eds.), *The genesis of language.* Cambridge: M.I.T. Press, 1966.

Menyuk, P. Syntactic rules used by children pre-school through first grade. *Journal of Child Development,* 1964, *35,* 533-546.

Menyuk, P. *Sentences children use.* Cambridge: M.I.T. Press, 1969.

Pipe, P. *Practical programming.* New York: Holt, Rinehart and Winston, 1966.

Sloane, H. and MacAulay, B. (Eds.) *Operant procedures in remedial speech and language training.* Boston: Houghton Mifflin Co., 1968.

Templin, M. *Certain language skills in children.* Minneapolis: The University of Minnesota Press, 1957.

Van Riper, C. *Speech correction: Principles and methods.* Englewood Cliffs, N. J.: Prentice-Hall, 1963.

3 Preparation

The purpose of this chapter is to set forth basic principles, procedures, and examples to prepare the teacher to carry out the language programs. There are three general areas: ancillary language training, behavior management, and the use of supportive personnel and equipment. Ancillary language training procedures refer to testing, charting, scoring, etc. Behavior management refers to general behaviors such as attending, sitting, looking, etc. The use of supportive personnel and equipment includes teacher-aides, parents, and teaching machines.

Ancillary Language Training Procedures

The language programs discussed in Chapter Two are the core of the language training program. There are additional activities which relate to the programs and aid in their successful use. These procedures include evaluation, measurement of language performance, recording data, the teaching setting, and parent carry-over. The purpose of this section is to discuss these procedures and present examples of them. An overview of the evaluation and measurement procedures is shown in Table 8.

Initial Evaluation

The first step is to select children who need language training. Historically, evaluation (diagnosis) has included a description of the problem, a case history to indicate possible causation, and extensive testing procedures to further describe and define the problem (Johnson, Darley, and Spriestersbach, 1963).

Table 8   Measurement Procedures and Use of Results

Test	Results Indicate
1 Evaluation	Need for Language Training
2 PCLT	Which Program
3 Criterion Test	Pre- and Post-Measure of Program
4 Placement	Where to Start in a Program
5 Show and Tell — School / Home	Carry-over of Language

Many language tests such as the Illinois Test of Psycholinguistic Ability (Kirk, McCarthy, and Kirk, 1968), the Houston Test for Language Development (Crabtree, 1958), the Northwestern Syntax Screening Test (Lee, 1969), the Peabody Picture Vocabulary Test (Dunn, 1959), portions of the Stanford-Binet (Terman and Merrill, 1960), and the Weschler Intelligence Scale for Children (Weschler, 1949) are commonly used by language teachers. A number of other language tests are found in the works of Bangs (1961), Carrow (1968), Englemann (1967), Lillywhite, et al. (1970), Zimmerman, Steiner, and Evatt (1969), Mecham, Jex, and Jones (1967), Johnson and Myklebust (1967), Berry (1969), and others. These tests all reflect the bias of their authors as to what constitutes normal language. Most of the tests cover a wide range of language abilities. Some of them, such as the Northwestern Syntax Screening Test, provide a measurement of only grammatical-syntactical language behavior.

Another form of testing is the collection of a sample of the child's natural, spontaneous language in a conversation with an interested adult. This sample may be collected in the home and/or clinic setting. The corpus can be analyzed to reveal grammatical-syntactical deficit using procedures described by Lee (1966), Lee and Canter (1971), Shriner (1967), Menyuk (1969), Bloom (1970), and others.

Any number of language tests may be administered for a wide variety of reasons. For the use of the language programs described in this book, the critical evaluation (diagnostic) question is "Does the child have an oral, expressive, language deficit?" This question may be answered simply by asking the parents and teachers about the child's talking and observing a small sample of his speech. If the child does demonstrate oral grammatical-syntactical deficit for his age, he is a candidate for the language training programs described in this book. To confirm this initial hypothesis and to decide whether or not the language programs will be useful, the teacher then gives the child the Programmed Conditioning for Language Test or PCLT.

PCLT

The Programmed Conditioning for Language Test, or PCLT, is a special test which measures the child's oral expressive language ability as circumscribed by the curriculum of the Programmed Conditioning for Language Programs. Hence, it is an internal test peculiar to the programs which measures what they teach. The test and directions for administering and scoring it are shown in Figure 18. The test is given in imitation form based on the observation that a child will repeat only what he can process (Lee, 1969; Menyuk, 1969).

In scoring the responses, the teacher should consider grammatical accuracy as the prime requisite. Semantic and articulatory deviations are permitted. The child may use any "words" to complete a sentence. These are scored as correct even though these may not be the exact words used in the stimulus utterance. For phonological variations the "words" must be intelligible approximations which are relatively consistent. The same rules for response evaluation (see Chapter Two) used in the program are used in the scoring of the PCLT.

The PCLT yields two scores. The Program Score indicates the number of programs (or grammatical forms) which the child already has. The Adequacy Score reflects the child's use of certain grammatical forms even though they are not entirely correct. The Program Score suggests the specific language training programs the child has or needs whereas the Adequacy Score gives an indication of his total expressive syntactical/grammatical language performance. The results of a pilot study to provide normative data about the PCLT for four- and five-year-old normal speaking children are shown in Table 9.

The four-year-old children were chosen from a private preschool nursery. There is a fairly large difference (15.2) between their Program Score (79.6) and the Adequacy Score (94.8). The Adequacy Score is a better indicator of their overall language ability whereas the Program Score indicates specific grammatical forms in error, commonly the omission of "the" and /s/ marker confusion. Of importance is the observation that most of the children scored 90 percent or better on the PCLT indicating that children four years of age are able to use the grammar contained in the mini-language taught in the program.

The five-year-old children were randomly selected from a group of 60 kindergarten-first grade children. Two children (both male) who demonstrated extremely low, deviate scores were excluded from the final sample. The majority of all the children scored above 90 percent on both measures. The most common errors were the omission of the word, "the," in the response, and /s/ marker confusion which accounted for most of the discrepancy between the Program Score and the Adequacy Score. It may be assumed from these data that the average

Figure 18   **PCLT Programmed Conditioning for Language Test**

PCLT

monterey language program

NAME _____

DATE _____ BIRTHDATE _____ AGE _____

PROGRAM SCORE _____ / 55 X 100 = _____ %

ADEQUACY SCORE _____ / 300 X 100 = _____ %

Draw a line through program items completely correct.   ( ) cumulative programs.

1 2 3 4 5 6 7 8 9 10 11 (12) 13 14 15 16 17 (18 19 20

21 22) 23 24 25 26 27 28 29 30 31 32 33 34 35 36 37 38 39 40

Test Item	Program Number and Score + or −	Adequacy Score Points	Test Item	Program Number and Score + or −	Adequacy Score Points
1. Identify 3 nouns	1	0	18. You are swimming in the water.	17	6
2. Say 3 nouns	2	3	19. They are looking at the man.	17	6
3. In the house.	3	3	20. We are standing by the boat.	17	6
4. The boy is in the yard.	4	6	21. The cat jumped on the table.	23	6
5. The dog is biting the bone.	5	6	22. The lady was driving the car.	24	6
6. Q Is the cat eating the food?	6	6	23. The birds were flying in the sky.	24	7
7. Q What is running in the grass?	7	6	24. Q Was the cat crying in the tree?	25	7
8. He is running on the ground.	8	6	25. Q Were the cars bumping the wall?	25	6
9. She is sitting in the chair.	8	6	26. Q What was the boy singing?	26	5
10. It is barking in the room.	8	6	27. Q What were the monkeys playing?	26	5
11. I am hitting the nail.	9	5	28. The man does jump in the hole.	27	7
12. The cat eats on the floor.	10	6	29. The cows do like the grass.	27	6
13. The boys run in the street.	11	6	30. The lady did eat by the car.	28	7
14. The man is walking in the yard.	13	7	31. Q Do the dogs bark?	29	4
15. The girls are walking in the grass.	14	7	32. Q Does the boy run?	29	4
16. Q Are the ladies sewing the shirt?	15	6	33. Q Did the airplane fly?	29	4
17. Q What are the dogs licking?	16	5	34. Q What is the girl doing?	30	5

FORM 103   DISTRIBUTED BY MONTEREY LEARNING SYSTEMS, INC. • 99 VIA ROBLES, MONTEREY, CALIFORNIA • ©1971, BEHAVIORAL SCIENCES INSTITUTE

five-year-old normal language speaking child can produce the syntactical-grammatical forms included in the PCLT. The five-year-old children scored higher than the four-year-old children.

A sample of nonlanguage children's performance on the PCLT is shown in Table 10.

Figure 18, continued

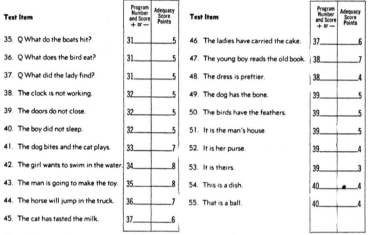

Test Item	Program Number and Score + or −	Adequacy Score Points	Test Item	Program Number and Score + or −	Adequacy Score Points
35. Q What do the boats hit?	31	5	46. The ladies have carried the cake.	37	6
36. Q What does the bird eat?	31	5	47. The young boy reads the old book.	38	7
37. Q What did the lady find?	31	5	48. The dress is preftier.	38	4
38. The clock is not working.	32	5	49. The dog has the bone.	39	5
39. The doors do not close.	32	5	50. The birds have the feathers.	39	5
40. The boy did not sleep.	32	5	51. It is the man's house.	39	5
41. The dog bites and the cat plays.	33	7	52. It is her purse.	39	4
42. The girl wants to swim in the water.	34	8	53. It is theirs.	39	3
43. The man is going to make the toy.	35	8	54. This is a dish.	40	4
44. The horse will jump in the truck.	36	7	55. That is a ball.	40	4
45. The cat has tasted the milk.	37	6			

Comments:

DIRECTIONS

ADMINISTRATION:

1. The child is to repeat each item after the examiner.
2. For statement test items say, "Say:_____"
3. For question test items (Q) say, "Ask me:_____?"
4. Administer each item only once.

SCORING:

1. There are two scores: 1) the Program Score which indicates the program language forms the child has and 2) the Adequacy Score which indicates the child's general syntactical adequacy as it relates to the language programs.
2. For the Program Score, score the entire sentence as either right or wrong. However, for test items 1-13, use only the **bold face** words to derive the score. For items 14-55, use all the words in the sentence. Add up the number of correct items to derive the Program Score.
3. For the Adequacy Score, score the entire sentence. Give a point for each correct word in the sentence.

Add up the number of points to derive the Adequacy Score.

4. Draw a line through the number of each program passed. Some of the programs are tested with several items. The child must pass all of the items to have a program scored as passed, e.g., items 8, 9, and 10 all refer to Program 8. The child must pass items 8, 9, and 10'to score a pass on Program 8.
5. Score contractions as correct, e.g. "he's", "gonna", "don't".
6. Score unintelligible or omitted responses wrong.
7. Score misarticulated, intelligible responses as correct.
8. Score substitutions of grammatically correct words as correct, e.g., No. 4: "The boy is in the yard." Response: "The girl is in the house."
9. Draw a line through omitted words.
10. Write in additional (don't score) or substituted words.

Materials: None, may use pictures or objects for item 1

85

Table 9   PCLT Program and Adequacy Scores
Expressed in Percentage for Two Groups
of Normal Speaking Children: Group A (N=17, 9 Female and
8 Male) and Group B (N=18, 9 Female and 9 Male).

	Item	Mean	S. D.	Median
Group A (N 17)				
	Age	4.6	.5	4.6
	Program	79.6	15.7	81.5
	Adequacy	94.8	4.8	96.3
Group B (N 18)				
	Age	5.6	.4	5.4
	Program	89.6	9.9	92.7
	Adequacy	96.7	3.5	98.4

Table 10   PCLT Program and Adequacy Scores
Expressed in Percentage for Two Groups
of Linguistically Divergent Children: Group A (N=11, 11 male)
and Group B (N=9, 5 male and 4 female).

	Item	Mean	S. D.	Median
Group A (N 11)				
	Age	4.8	.8	4.7
	Program	7.0	8.0	3.6
	Adequacy	41.0	25.0	28.0
Group B (N 9)				
	Age	6.3	1.5	6.0
	Program	41.5	31.6	41.8
	Adequacy	73.4	24.7	82.4

These data indicate that older nonlanguage children score lower on the PCLT than younger, normal speaking children. These children demonstrate a serious expressive language problem, as measured by the PCLT, when compared to a group of normal speaking children. Hence, it may be assumed that the PCLT does measure grammatical-syntactical ability and that it differentiates between normal speaking children and nonlanguage children.

The basic purpose of the PCLT is to tell the teacher which of the programs the child needs and where to place the child in the curriculum. Experience with the PCLT over the past eight years indicates that it accurately places children in the curriculum, exceptions to this are the echolalic child and the bilingual child. These children are skilled at imitation and may score high on the PCLT when in reality their daily use of the language forms is very limited. A simple way to overcome this diagnostic problem is to administer all of the criterion tests discussed in the following section in addition to the PCLT. These criterion test scores may then be used to measure the child's language ability for placement in the curriculum. Once the child is in the program, the criterion tests will be administered for each successive program regardless of his score on the PCLT. The reason for this is that children vary greatly in their imitative ability as a function of age and language ability. It is possible that a child who could pass PCLT items could not, or does not, use the form in his natural speech. The criterion tests are more difficult and measure the child's ability to produce a language form in response to questions thus approximating the spontaneous normal speaking situation. The PCLT should be readministered at regular intervals (quarterly) to measure the child's overall growth in language and as an overall post-test of language performance as taught by the programs.

After the PCLT has indicated which programs the child needs, the first failed program is located. The child is started on that program. For example, if the first failed program is No. 4 (Is), the child is started on that program. The child may experience some difficulty because he must learn both the program protocol and the correct response. Once in the program sequence the child continues to go from program to program taking the criterion test for each program.

Criterion Tests

Before starting a program, the child is given a criterion test to determine the adequacy of his performance for the particular grammatical form to be taught. The response evaluation is the same as for the PCLT and the language programs (see Chapter Two). The criterion test consists of questions which are asked to evoke the desired response. No social or token reinforcement is given during the criterion test. The questions take two forms: (1) "Wh" questions, such as "What color is the dog?" and (2) choice questions, such as "Is the dog brown or white? " When a child is beginning language program training, the choice question form is used more often. As the child becomes more competent in the use of language, the "Wh" questions are used more frequently. The teacher should use pictures or objects with the questions.

Suggested sample questions are shown in Figure 19 (see also the question or command series in each program). The teacher should use different words in each question and/or ask different questions for each child. The child is presented with five questions, like the examples, and his answers scored accordingly. The number of correct responses is divided by the total number of questions and multiplied by 100 to derive a percentage correct response score on the criterion test.

Example: $\dfrac{\text{number correct}}{\text{total}}$ X 100 = _____ % correct

$$\frac{4}{5} \text{ X } 100 = 80\% \text{ correct}$$

Figure 19   Criterion Test Sample Questions

These are sample questions and responses for the criterion tests. They have been selected from the question series in each program. See the question series in each program for the specific question forms and responses desired. Score only the underlined terms. Substitution of grammatically appropriate words and/or intelligible misarticulations are permitted. Use pictures or objects.
Present five questions for most programs.
Score = $\dfrac{\text{number correct}}{5}$ X 100 or percentage correct.

In programs 8, 17, 23, 25, 28, 32-36, 38, 39 and the cumulative programs (18, 19, 20, 21, and 22) present 15 questions and score $\dfrac{\text{number correct}}{15}$ X 100 or percentage correct.

Administer criterion tests before the program and after the program has been completed. Use Criterion Test Score Record form.

Program Number	Name	Question	Response
1	Identification of nouns	Touch the ball.	Child touches ball.
2	Naming nouns	What is this?	Noun
3	In/on	Where is the ball?	in the house
4	Is	Is the ball round or square?	The ball is round.
		Where is the tree?	The tree is in the yard.
5	Is verbing	Is the boy walking or running?	The boy is walking.
		or	
		What is the girl holding?	The girl is holding a pen.
		or	
		Where is the dog sleeping?	The dog is sleeping on the floor.
6	Is interrogative	Guess if the ball is round or square?	Is the ball round?
		or	

		Guess if the toy is on the shelf or on the floor?	Is the toy on the shelf?
		or	
		Guess if the girl is walking or running?	Is the girl running?
		or	
		Guess if the boy is playing in the water or snow?	Is the boy playing in the snow?
7	What is	I see something big, ask me what.	What is big?
		or	
		Something is in the house, ask me what.	What is in the house?
		or	
		Something is moving in the grass, ask me what.	What is moving in the grass?
		or	
		The girl is holding something, ask me what.	What is the girl holding?
8	He/she/it	Is (he/she/it) big or little?	(He/she/it) is big.
		or	
		What is (he/she/it) holding?	(He/she/it) is holding money.
		or	
		Where is (he/she/it) standing?	(He/she/it) is standing on the floor.
9	I am	Are you a boy or a girl?	I am a boy.
		or	
		Where are you?	I am in school.
		or	
		What are you wearing?	I am wearing shoes.
		or	
		Where are you hiding?	I am hiding in the closet.
10	Singular noun present tense	What does the man hold?	The man holds the ball.
		or	
		Where does the man work?	The man works in the yard.
		or	
		Does the girl stand or sit?	The girl stands.
11	Plural nouns present tense	Do the boys walk or run?	The boys run.
		or	
		What do the girls throw?	The girls throw stones.
		or	
		Where do the dogs run?	The dogs run in the yard.
12	Cumulative plural-singular present tense	(Programs 11 and 12)	

Figure 19, continued

Program Number	Name	Question	Response
13	The	Where is the boy?	The boy is in the yard.
		or	
		What is the girl holding?	The girl is holding the doll.
14	Plural nouns are	Are the boys nice or mean?	The boys are nice.
		or	
		What are the boys kicking?	The boys are kicking the ball.
15	Are interrogative	Guess if the girls are tall or short?	Are the girls tall?
		or	
		Guess if the trees are in the grass or in the dirt?	Are the tress in the grass?
		or	
		Guess if the boys are holding a ball or a book?	Are the boys holding a ball?
		or	
		Guess if the flowers are growing in the house or in the garden?	Are the flowers growing in the house?
16	What are	The boys are catching something, ask me what.	What are the boys catching?
		or	
		The boys are kicking something in the grass, ask me what.	What are the boys kicking in the grass?
17	You/they/we	Where am I sitting?	You are sitting in a chair.
		or	
		What am I wearing?	You are wearing a dress.
		or	
		Where are they playing?	They are playing on the floor.
		or	
		What are they holding?	They are holding a book.
		or	
		What are we sharing?	We are sharing the toy.
		or	
		Where are we looking?	We are looking in the mirror.
18	Cumulative pronouns	(Programs 8, 9, and 17)	
19	Cumulative is/are/am	(Programs 4, 5, 6, 8, and 9)	
20	Cumulative is/are/am interrogative	(Programs 6, 15 plus pronouns from 8, 9, and 17)	
21	Cumulative what is/are/am	(Programs 7, 16 plus pronouns from 8, 9, and 17)	

22	Cumulative noun/pronoun// verb/verbing	(Programs 5, 8, 9, 10, 11, 14, and 17)	
23	Singular and plural past tense	What did the boy play?	The boy played ball.
		or	
		Where did the girls jump?	The girls jumped in the air.
24	Was/were	Was the girl happy or sad?	The girl was happy.
		or	
		What was the dog chasing?	The dog was chasing the cat.
		or	
		Where was the plane flying?	The plane was flying in the sky.
		(Same for plurals and were)	
25	Was/were interrogative	Guess if the boy was mean or nice?	Was the boy mean?
		or	
		Guess if the girl was in school or at home?	Was the girl in school?
		or	
		Guess if the baby was drinking milk or juice?	Was the baby drinking milk?
		or	
		Guess if the man was resting in the chair or in the bed?	Was the man resting?
		(Same for plural and were)	
26	What was/ were	The boy was hiding something, ask me what.	What was the boy hiding?
		or	
		Something was big, ask me what.	What was big?
		or	
		Something was flying in the air, ask me what.	What was flying in the air?
		(Same for plural and what were)	
27	Does/do	Does the dog run or walk?	The dog does run.
		or	
		Does the girl play ball or house?	The girl does play house.
		or	
		Do the trees grow or die?	The trees do grow.
		or	
		Do the dogs eat bones or hay?	The dogs do eat bones.
28	Did	Did the girl skip or dance?	The girl did skip.
		or	
		Did the cat run fast or slow?	The cat did run fast.

Program Number	Name	Question	Response
		or	
		What did the baby eat?	The baby did eat food.
		or	
		Where did the planes land?	The planes did land on the ground.
29	Do/does/did interrogative	Guess, do the boys walk or run?	Do the boys walk?
		or	
		Guess, does the man run on the ground or in the air?	Does the man run on the ground?
		or	
		Guess, did the dog sleep or eat in the house?	Did the dog eat in the house?
30	What is/are doing	The boy is doing something, ask me what.	What is the boy doing?
		or	
		The wheels are doing something, ask me what.	What are the wheels doing?
31	What do/does/did	The boy hits something, ask me what.	What does the boy hit?
		or	
		The girls play something, ask me what.	What do the girls play?
		or	
		Mommy cooked something, ask me what?	What did mommy cook?
32	Negative not	Is the boy sad?	The boy is not sad.
		or	
		Are the trees dying?	The trees are not dying.
		or	
		Does the food spoil?	The food does not spoil.
		or	
		Did the girl win?	The girl did not win.
33	Conjunction and	Does the girl walk and run or skip and hop?	The girl walks and runs.
		or	
		Do the boys and girls play or the dogs and the cats?	The dogs and the cats play.
		or	
		Do the baby and the mommy play and rest or eat and drink?	The baby and the mommy eat and drink.
		or	
		Do the boys walk and the girls run or the girls walk and the boys run?	The girls walk and the boys run.

34	Infinitive to	Does the boy need to walk or to run?	The boy needs to walk.
		or	
		Where does the girl like to play?	The girl likes to play in the yard.
		or	
		What do the friends want to drink?	The friends want to drink the milk.
35	Future tense to	What is the girl going to eat?	The girl is going to eat candy.
		or	
		Where are the boys going to play?	The boys are going to play on the carpet.
		or	
		Where is the man going?	The man is going to the house.
36	Future tense will	What will the baby wear?	The baby will wear pajamas.
		or	
		Where will the cats sleep?	The cats will sleep in the bed.
37	Perfect tense	Have the trees blossomed or died?	The trees have blossomed.
		or	
		Has the boy laughed or cried?	The boy has cried.
		or	
		Has the girl walked the dog or the cat?	The girl has walked the dog.
38	Adjectives	Is the picture bigger or smaller?	This picture is smaller.
		or	
		Which tree is the tallest?	That tree is the tallest.
		or	
		Does the blue car or the green car run?	The blue car runs.
39	Possessives	Is it the boy's or girl's?	It is the boy's.
		or	
		Is it yours or mine?	It is mine.
		or	
		Does the boy have the ball or the truck?	The boy has the ball.
		or	
		Is it the boy's truck or the girl's truck?	It is the boy's truck.
		or	
		Is it my truck or your truck?	It is my truck.
40	This/that/a	What is this?	This is a ball.
		or	
		What is that?	That is a tree.

Figure 19, continued

Program Number	Name	Question	Response
41	Articulation Program	Any question to evoke target word or target word in a sentence	target word alone or in a sentence

The criterion test questions reflect the forms taught in a program such as "The subject verbs preposition the noun." The longer or longest forms are chosen to provide an adequate test. In program No. 8 (He/She/It), No. 17 (You/They/We), and No. 28 (Do/Does/Did) five questions for each form are asked; hence in these programs the criterion test consists of 15 items, five from each of the forms.

In the cumulative programs (No. 18, 19, 20, 21, and 22) and for programs No. 23, 25, 32-36, 38, and 39, the teacher should also use 15 questions which are selected from the various forms in these programs. In the administration of the criterion test the teacher should take care to mix the grammatical forms.

Example: $\dfrac{\text{number correct}}{\text{total}} \times 100 = \underline{\hspace{2cm}}$ % correct

$$\frac{10}{15} \times 100 = 66\% \text{ correct}$$

The scores of the criterion test are used to determine whether or not a child should go through the program and to measure his performance before and after the program. If a child scores 80 percent or above on his before program criterion test, he does not need the program and should move on to the next program. If the child scores below 80 percent on the before criterion test, he is put through the program. The form for recording the criterion test is shown in Figure 20. The child's response should be written in and scored right or wrong.

The criterion test is readministered with no social or token reinforcement after the child has completed the program. It is recommended that the after criterion test be administered the day following the child's completion of a program in order to provide an appropriate test of his proficiency in the use of the form.

Figure 20   Criterion Test Recording Form

CRITERION TEST

monterey language program

NAME _____

PROGRAM _____

COMMENTS _____

_____

☐ BEFORE PROGRAM   DATE_____ %_____

1. _____

2. _____

3. _____

4. _____

5. _____

☐ AFTER PROGRAM   DATE_____ %_____

1. _____

2. _____

3. _____

4. _____

5. _____

FORM 105   DISTRIBUTED BY MONTEREY LEARNING SYSTEMS, INC. • 99 VIA ROBLES, MONTEREY, CALIFORNIA • ©1971, BEHAVIORAL SCIENCES INSTITUTE

If a child scores below 80 percent on the *after* criterion test, he should be recycled through the last three series of the program and the criterion test readministered. If he does not score higher on the second administration of the *after* criterion test, he should be moved on to the next program because commonly, the same forms will be presented again in subsequent programs. Children occasionally fail the *after* criterion test during early programs because they have not yet mastered the ability to transfer the form to the more spontaneous criterion test setting. As they proceed through various programs, this transfer skill will be increased. In addition, the teacher can continue to evoke and reinforce these forms during the show and tell period. The criterion test scores are recorded to document the child's progress and accumulation of language forms.

Show and Tell

A simple, convenient way of providing for transfer of training and obtaining a sample of spontaneous language is to hold a brief "Show and Tell" period during each training session. During this period the child can talk about some object or picture. The teacher attempts to evoke ten sentences from each child and may ask questions to elicit specific language forms which the child has just learned. Criterion tests may also be administered during this period. A list of the programs each child has completed and the criterion test questions are helpful to the teacher in conducting the show and tell period. The teacher also may ask other kinds of questions, make statements, or merely keep quiet in order to evoke language from the child. Techniques described by Muma (1970) would be appropriate during this period. Only social reinforcement is used.

The child's responses are recorded on the Spontaneous Language Record Form shown in Figure 21. One child's spontaneous language responses may be recorded over several sessions with a new date for each session, or a group of children's spontaneous responses may be shown for one session. The teacher may scan the Spontaneous Language Record Form to quickly determine whether the children are transferring their newly learned forms to the more spontaneous show and tell language situation.

Two other more formal analyses are also helpful. The first type recognizes the percentages of single words, phrases, and sentences utilized. It is expected that children will use proportionately more words and phrases when they start the language training program

Figure 21 Spontaneous Language Recording Form

SPONTANEOUS LANGUAGE RECORD

monterey language program

DATE ____________________

NAME	SINGLE WORDS	PHRASES	SENTENCES

FORM 107 DISTRIBUTED BY MONTEREY LEARNING SYSTEMS, INC. • 99 VIA ROBLES, MONTEREY, CALIFORNIA • ©1971, BEHAVIORAL SCIENCES INSTITUTE

and more sentences after they have improved in language. The percentage of each of these may be computed and compared.

Example:

$$\frac{\text{number of single word utterances}}{\text{total utterances}} \times 100 = \underline{\quad}\% \text{ of single words}$$

$$\frac{\text{number of phrase utterances}}{\text{total utterances}} \times 100 = \underline{\quad}\% \text{ of phrase utterances}$$

$$\frac{\text{number of sentence utterances}}{\text{total utterances}} \times 100 = \underline{\quad}\% \text{ of sentence utterances}$$

$$\frac{7}{10} \times 100 = 70\% \text{ words or phrases or sentences}$$

Another type of analysis would compute the number of grammatically correct sentences.

Example:

$$\frac{\text{number of grammatically correct sentences}}{\text{total number of sentences}} \times 100 = \underline{\quad}\% \text{ of correct sentences}$$

$$\frac{3}{5} \times 100 = 60\% \text{ correct sentences}$$

The scoring rules are the same as for the PCLT and/or language programs themselves. The child who has not been taught "the" in the language programs could not be expected to use it in spontaneous language. The percentage of words, phrases, and sentences and the percentage of correct sentences can be computed per child or per group of children. This computation should be made at regular calendar intervals such as weekly, biweekly, or monthly. Show and tell may be viewed as a speech setting which is less formal than the programs, but more formal than spontaneous language settings in the home or school. This information yields a measurement of the transfer of training and the efficiency of the program in improving the children's natural, spontaneous language performance.

Spontaneous Language Samples

The critical evidence of language skills is the use of the appropriate grammatical forms in spontaneous language in home, social, and school settings. The basic procedure is to listen to the child in these environments and record his spontaneous language. The recording form shown for use during show and tell time may be employed, or the teacher may merely collect a list of sentences spoken by the child during the observation period. It is helpful to tape record this observation. Lee and

Canter (1971) suggest that samples collected when the children are interacting with an adult demonstrate better language performance than those taken of the child talking with other children. Our own experience has been similar. Furthermore, we have found that samples taken in the school environment have paralleled samples taken from the home environment.

The language corpus may then be submitted to analysis. The same procedures used for analyzing the sample taken during show and tell may be used, or the teacher may wish to use other procedures such as those suggested by Lee and Canter (1971), Shriner (1969), Miner (1969), and Menyuk (1969). Of particular interest is the child's use of the forms taught in the language programs, or his mini-language, and what new forms he has generated on his own during the mini-language. As another casual measurement of spontaneous language adequacy, the child may be observed in a typical school environment for a period of time and the classroom teacher questioned as to her opinion of his oral language adequacy. If he "sounds all right" or "no different from the other children," we may assume that he has met the test of appropriate oral language. This same gross, but practical, measurement of language adequacy may also be employed with the parent.

Although somewhat difficult to obtain and analyze, samples of spontaneous language collected in environments other than the training setting yield important information about the adequacy of the training programs. The teacher should develop procedures for collecting and analyzing spontaneous language samples. These should be conducted at regular intervals during the calendar year, e.g., monthly, quarterly, etc.

Scoring and Timing

When a child is working on a program, the teacher evaluates and scores each of his responses. The score sheet to be used is shown in Figure 22. The child's name is to be placed to the left of the score spaces (1-40). It is possible to use the same score sheet for one child over several sessions or to place several different children's names on the same score sheet for one session. The program should be named, the criterion indicated (commonly it is ten or twenty), the date of the session, and the time spent in the session. All of this information goes in the upper right hand corner. The program step is written next to the child's name. If several children are being scored on one sheet, each child's name, program name, and step (also criterion, if appropriate) is written in the left hand column opposite the score spaces. Usually, the children will spend approximately the same amount of time in the program each day; hence, one notation on time will be sufficient.

Figure 22 **Score Sheet**

SCORE SHEET

monterey language program

NAME________________________________

PROGRAM________________ CRITERION__________

DATE________________________________

MIN. PER SESSION______ GROUP/INDIVIDUAL__________

1	2	3	4	5	6	7	8	9	10	11	12	13	14	15	16	17	18	19	20	TOTALS
																				X/____
21	22	23	24	25	26	27	28	29	30	31	32	33	34	35	36	37	38	39	40	X/O____
																				%____
1	2	3	4	5	6	7	8	9	10	11	12	13	14	15	16	17	18	19	20	
																				X/____
21	22	23	24	25	26	27	28	29	30	31	32	33	34	35	36	37	38	39	40	X/O____
																				%____
1	2	3	4	5	6	7	8	9	10	11	12	13	14	15	16	17	18	19	20	
																				X/____
21	22	23	24	25	26	27	28	29	30	31	32	33	34	35	36	37	38	39	40	X/O____
																				%____
1	2	3	4	5	6	7	8	9	10	11	12	13	14	15	16	17	18	19	20	
																				X/____
21	22	23	24	25	26	27	28	29	30	31	32	33	34	35	36	37	38	39	40	X/O____
																				%____
1	2	3	4	5	6	7	8	9	10	11	12	13	14	15	16	17	18	19	20	
																				X/____
21	22	23	24	25	26	27	28	29	30	31	32	33	34	35	36	37	38	39	40	X/O____
																				%____
1	2	3	4	5	6	7	8	9	10	11	12	13	14	15	16	17	18	19	20	
																				X/____
21	22	23	24	25	26	27	28	29	30	31	32	33	34	35	36	37	38	39	40	X/O____
																				%____

KEY: X=CORRECT AND REINFORCED /=CORRECT BUT NOT REINFORCED 0=INCORRECT

FORM 101 DISTRIBUTED BY MONTEREY LEARNING SYSTEMS, INC. • 99 VIA ROBLES, MONTEREY, CALIFORNIA • ©1971, BEHAVIORAL SCIENCES INSTITUTE

Example: Mary J.
           A3

	1	2	3	4	5

           10

	21	22	23	24	25

           3/10/71

After the child has made his response, the teacher has evaluated the response and administered the reinforcer, the child's response is scored on the score sheet.

Example:

X right and reinforced with token and "Good"

| X | | | | | | | |

/ right and reinforced with "Good" only

| / | | | | | | | |

0 wrong

| 0 | | | | | | | |

NR No Response (do not score right or wrong but write in NR above the square. NR's are not calculated.)

NR

| | | | | | | | |

Unintelligible   Nothing

After a session, the total number of responses and the number of correct responses are counted for each child. The number correct is then divided by the total number and multiplied by 100 to yield a percentage of correctness.

Example:

$$\frac{\text{number correct (X \& /) X 100}}{\text{total (X, / and 0)}} = \underline{\hspace{2cm}}\text{\% correct}$$

$$\frac{10 = (6 \text{ and } 4) \text{ X } 100}{15 = (6, 4 \text{ and } 5)} = 66.7\% \text{ correct}$$

Criterion. The criterion of performance was discussed in Chapter Two, but it is presented here again to show its determination during the scoring process. Criterion refers to the number of successive correct responses a child must emit before he can go on to the next step. Or put another way, criterion refers to the number of successive "X's" and "/'s" not interrupted by a zero. This is indicated by a slash mark.

Example:

Criterion	Child's score	Meets criterion

Criterion 10

1	2	3	4	5	6	7	8	9	10	11	12	13	14	15	16
X	0	0	/	0	X	X	X	/	X	/	X	X	/	X	

   In group training the criterion is commonly ten. If the child is working alone or with only one other child, the criterion is doubled. This is done to prevent the child from moving through the program too fast. When the child has met criterion on a step, he then goes on to the next step. If a child has not completed the criterion performance for a step in one session, he must start over again in the next session. For example, if the child has achieved seven successive correct responses in Monday's session, he would have to start over and score ten more successively correct in Tuesday's session.

Charting. A chart to record percentages is used continuously along with the programs. The chart is shown in Figure 23. Information including the child's name, the criterion, before and after criterion test scores, the program name and number, the date, minutes per session, and whether or not the child was working with a group or individually is written in the spaces indicated in the lower left hand portion of the chart. The actual steps the child covered in each session (Series A, Step 1, Series A, Step 2, etc.) are listed at the bottom of the chart for each session.

   The percentage correct, the total number of responses, and the actual steps covered in each session are posted on the chart each day. The lower part of the chart is divided into 0-100 percent for percent of correct responses. The upper part of the chart shows the total number of responses for each session, 0-160.

   If Johnny scored 86 percent in session one, 81 percent in session two, 87 percent in session three, 82 percent in session four, and 90 percent in session five, his responses would be put on the chart as illustrated. These scores are entered as dots and con-

Figure 23   **Chart**

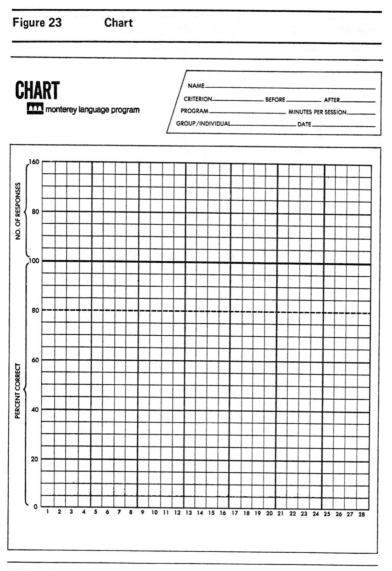

nected by straight lines. If he responded 40, 50, 45, 35, and 60 times for each of the five sessions, respectively, they would be recorded as dots in the upper part and connected. The dotted line at 80 percent is to call the teacher's attention to the percentage of accuracy level which indicates the need for branching.

Figure 24   Five Types of Chart Configurations

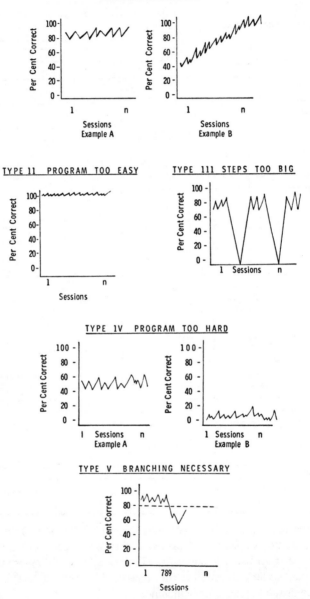

The charting process provides some additional information which makes it possible to visibly and graphically portray the efficiency of the programs. There are several charting configurations which have special meaning and can be helpful to the teacher. These are shown in Figure 24.

The most common type of chart (Type I) is the normal run chart. Note that there is some variation between steps and series, but the overall run will be between 75 percent and 100 percent accuracy. In early programs, there will also be a fairly low performance initially as the child learns new form in the first series. There may also be dips at the beginning of each series. Gradually, he will improve throughout the program and his overall average will be 90 percent or better.

A Type II configuration indicates that the program is probably too easy and the child really doesn't need it. This is a fairly common chart, however, for echolalic or non-English speaking children. They will eventually show dips in percentage correct in the question, command, story, and conversation series.

The Type III configuration means the steps are too big, especially between series. The child learns the form, but only after some difficulty in the early steps in a series. If this persists for either given children or programs, additional steps may be necessary to increase their percentage correct or to improve the program. These additional steps are referred to as "inserts." It might be important to go to the BI, especially the 250-257 series, in order to gradually build these new responses by backward chaining methods.

In a Type IV chart configuration, the response accuracy remains in the 40-60 percent range. This indicates that the child never quite mastered the response to the initial series or to the first step. The initial response was not so difficult that the child failed completely, but it was of sufficient difficulty to cause incomplete mastery. The only remedy for this situation is to write a series to precede series A, step I. If this is not done, the response accuracy will remain in the 40-60 percent range and the child will not acquire the target performance.

A Type V is the branching configuration where response accuracy drops to under 80 percent for three days. This indicates the necessity for instituting branching procedures. The charts themselves have a dashed line at 80 percent so it is very clear when the response accuracy drops under this percentage.

These are the basic chart configurations. It is important to keep the charts up to date. The information on the charts represents a convenient summary for any given child's performance. The information may also be collated to show a group's performance either on one language program or a set of them.

Initiate Home Carryover, IHC

At the end of each program (except for program No. 1), the symbols, IHC, are found. These stand for Initiate Home Carryover. As the child completes each program, his parents are asked to engage in carryover activities. They are given a form which gives them instructions on what to do, the responses expected, dates, times, and a score sheet. This form is shown in Figure 25.

Let us assume that a child has completed the "Is" (No. 4) program. Examples of the language constructions, "Boy is old," "Girl is in house," are written on the IHC form so that the parents may know exactly what the child can do. They are further instructed to find pictures in magazines or catalogues and go through them asking questions, such as "Is the car new or old?", "Where is the dog?" These are the same forms of questions which were on the language programs. The parents are to evaluate the child's responses and score them either "/" (correct) or "0" (incorrect). The parents are to give only social reinforcement like "Good," "That's right," etc. for correct responses and to simply repeat the sentence correctly for incorrect responses.

They are to do this for eight days for approximately five to ten minutes a day within a two-week period. They are asked to return the IHC form. This minimal parent activity has produced adequate transfer of training as reported by the mothers and noted in home observations. By the time the parents are asked to work with the child, he is quite capable of producing the desired responses correctly. Parents vary in their ability to complete home carryover activities. Occasionally, further instructions or requests to finish the IHC procedures are necessary.

The home carryover program is started prior to the final criterion test because most children pass the final criterion test at a higher percentage than the entering one, occasionally a child will not. The home carryover program usually is successful even with these children. However, the teacher might want to monitor a specific child's behavior and give the criterion test to assure readiness prior to the home carryover program.

Figure 25   Home Carry Over Form

HOME CARRY OVER RECORD FORM

monterey language program

NAME_____
INSTRUCTION _____
LANGUAGE CONSTRUCTION_____
EXAMPLES_____

DATE:
TIME PERIOD:
COMMENTS:

1	2	3	4	5	6	7	8	9	10	11	12	13	14	15	16	17
18	19	20	21	22	23	24	25	26	27	28	29	30	31	32	33	34
35	36	37	38	39	40	41	42	43	44	45	46	47	48	49	50	51

DATE:
TIME PERIOD:
COMMENTS:

1	2	3	4	5	6	7	8	9	10	11	12	13	14	15	16	17
18	19	20	21	22	23	24	25	26	27	28	29	30	31	32	33	34
35	36	37	38	39	40	41	42	43	44	45	46	47	48	49	50	51

DATE:
TIME PERIOD:
COMMENTS:

1	2	3	4	5	6	7	8	9	10	11	12	13	14	15	16	17
18	19	20	21	22	23	24	25	26	27	28	29	30	31	32	33	34
35	36	37	38	39	40	41	42	43	44	45	46	47	48	49	50	51

DATE:
TIME PERIOD:
COMMENTS:

1	2	3	4	5	6	7	8	9	10	11	12	13	14	15	16	17
18	19	20	21	22	23	24	25	26	27	28	29	30	31	32	33	34
35	36	37	38	39	40	41	42	43	44	45	46	47	48	49	50	51

DATE:
TIME PERIOD:
COMMENTS:

1	2	3	4	5	6	7	8	9	10	11	12	13	14	15	16	17
18	19	20	21	22	23	24	25	26	27	28	29	30	31	32	33	34
35	36	37	38	39	40	41	42	43	44	45	46	47	48	49	50	51

DATE:
TIME PERIOD:
COMMENTS:

1	2	3	4	5	6	7	8	9	10	11	12	13	14	15	16	17
18	19	20	21	22	23	24	25	26	27	28	29	30	31	32	33	34
35	36	37	38	39	40	41	42	43	44	45	46	47	48	49	50	51

DATE:
TIME PERIOD:
COMMENTS:

1	2	3	4	5	6	7	8	9	10	11	12	13	14	15	16	17
18	19	20	21	22	23	24	25	26	27	28	29	30	31	32	33	34
35	36	37	38	39	40	41	42	43	44	45	46	47	48	49	50	51

DATE:
TIME PERIOD:
COMMENTS:

1	2	3	4	5	6	7	8	9	10	11	12	13	14	15	16	17
18	19	20	21	22	23	24	25	26	27	28	29	30	31	32	33	34
35	36	37	38	39	40	41	42	43	44	45	46	47	48	49	50	51

/=CORRECT   O=INCORRECT

FORM 106   DISTRIBUTED BY MONTEREY LEARNING SYSTEMS, INC. • 99 VIA ROBLES, MONTEREY, CALIFORNIA • ©1971, BEHAVIORAL SCIENCES INSTITUTE

Individual vs. Group Structure

The programs basically involve an interaction between the teacher and the child. The common criterion level is ten. When the programs are being run with less than three children, the criterion is doubled. In the group setting it is possible for each of the children to be on a different program. Running the programs in a group requires skill on the part of the teacher. Experience has shown that a trained teacher can manage groups of up to seven in number.

There are two major and a number of minor considerations which concern group vs. individual teaching settings. The first major factor is defined as the acceleration hypothesis. There is evidence that when children move too quickly through programs they tend not to hold the response (the newly acquired language form). It is hypothesized that this is because they have not had an opportunity to really master the new form nor be exposed to it enough times in their natural environment.

When a child is seen alone or with one other child for sessions of twenty minutes or longer, there is danger of overacceleration occurring. In larger groups, there is less danger of this. A group of six children seen for one hour would result in about ten minutes of training for each child. Thus, the likelihood of overacceleration occurring is substantially reduced. To help control this problem, the language programs double the criterion for passing a step from ten to twenty successively correct responses whenever a child is seen alone or with one other child. This has the effect of reducing the number of steps which he can pass in a session.

The second major factor is defined as the modelling hypothesis. There is much evidence to support the notion that children learn from observing other children learn (Bandura, 1969). In the large group setting (six to seven children), each of the children may be on a different program. They are being exposed to, although not required to respond to, a wide variety of different language forms. They may learn much from these observations of other children going through more complex language programs. It has not yet been possible to isolate and measure this factor in the language programs. It undoubtedly interacts with the acceleration hypothesis. Thus far, our experience shows no difference in percentage correct or number of responses to complete a program between group and individual training.

A minor consideration in the group vs. individual decision is the mechanical problem of the administration and scoring of several programs for several children. This is possible for one teacher to do but not practical because of low response rates. However, the teacher can administer a number of programs at once if someone else does the scoring.

Another minor consideration is the management of children with unusual behavior problems. Our experience has shown that these children can be controlled more effectively by putting them in a group or with another child who is behaving appropriately. There is both a modeling effect and an opportunity to ignore (time out) the misbehaving child while the teacher works with the other child. This effect is especially powerful in a group of six or seven children.

A final minor consideration concerns the setting of the therapy activity. We are unable to recommend the ideal setting. The language programs will run in both individual and group settings. When research has yielded more information about the acceleration and modeling hypotheses, it should be possible to make more specific recommendations. Until that time, individual teachers will have to assess their own situation and their own goals for the children with whom they are working. Fortunately, the language programs will run in many different settings.

Length of Sessions

Programs have been run in varying time periods from two 30-minute periods a week to 90 minutes a day, five days a week. The age of the child is important. Although it has been possible, using powerful behavioral management systems, to get three-year-old children to attend to language learning for up to 90 minutes, this time period is not especially recommended. The children do fatigue.

The most important factor is the severity of the child's language problem as measured by the number of language programs he needs to complete. If the average nonlanguage child takes 3.7 hours per program and needs an average 11 programs to develop mini-syntax and grammar, the teacher must consider a minimum of 40 hours of training time. A child who takes ten hours per program and needs 20 programs will require 200 hours of language training time.

There are little data on the optimal time period or frequency of contact. We can only share our observations about the programs and our experience with the average time and number of programs per child. The teachers will have to examine their teaching loads, goals, and settings to determine their length of training sessions. The programs will run successfully within broad time limits.

Behavior Management

Before and during the language training it is important that the child is prepared to attend to the task of learning to talk. This is a simple truism that any teacher knows. The teacher must have the child's interest and attention before the child can learn anything. Most children have developed some competency early in life to maintain an attention span; however, many nonlanguage children have not—partly due to their language deficit and partly due to the same factors which produced it. The procedures to be described below may be necessary for only a few of the children the teacher will encounter. The experienced teacher must discern between the child who needs little or no behavior management and one who needs a great deal. It is efficient, good teaching to apply the procedures only when they are necessary. They will be mandatory with hyperactive, inattentive children.

The basic principle of behavior management is that behavior is determined by the stimuli which evoke it and the consequences which follow it (Skinner, 1953; Bandura, 1969; Ullman and Krasner, 1965; Patterson and Gullion, 1968; Yates, 1970). Stimuli which precede and summon behavior include such things as teachers, materials, and instructions. These set the stage for the child to behave. Consequences which follow behavior include such events as attention, "Good," and tokens which can be exchanged for toys. These affect the probability that the behavior will occur again. In order to manage the child's behavior, the teacher must carefully define the behavior—first for himself or herself and later for the child. The teacher can manipulate the stimuli and consequences which determine the occurrence of the behavior. These principles can be used to develop a behavior management system.

The behavior management system described in the following pages was developed over the past eight years at Children's House, evolving from work with the children there. There are many such strategies possible (Haring and Lovitt, 1967; Haring and Phillips, 1962; Ullman and Krasner, 1965; Hewitt, 1968; Walker, Mattson, and Buckley, 1969). This is only one possible system.

Defining Behaviors

A critical first step in behavior management is the definition of both desired and undesired behaviors. This definition must be in terms of a clearly observable event. The teacher must be able to consistently detect both the behavior's presence and its absence. A list of behaviors may be made which includes both the desired behaviors and their undesired correlates. At Children's House 34 positive behaviors and their opposites were defined and listed. Those six behaviors which pertain to language training time only are shown below:

Desired	Undesired
sits at desk	runs around room
attends to teacher	looks around room
keeps hands quiet	moves hands noisily
keeps feet quiet	moves feet noisily
responds to program stimulus	no response to program stimulus
waits quietly and attentively for turn	talks out of turn and doesn't attend to teacher

With such a list of behaviors, the teacher may determine stimuli which evoke them and consequences which affect their frequency. Both desired and undesired behaviors may be counted and their occurrence recorded to detect the effects of the controlling stimuli and consequences.

Stimulus Manipulation

One method of managing behavior is to present appropriate stimuli, commonly instructions, to evoke the desired behavior. It is best to concentrate on desirable behavior and try to set the stage for its occurrence. In the Children's House program, we found that fifteen such instructions were adequate to evoke the desired behavior patterns. A sample of five of these instructions pertaining to language training time follows:

Instructions	Desired Behaviors
"Show me you are ready"	Sits quietly looking at teacher
"Sit at your desk"	with hands folded on the desk
"Make your feet quiet"	top and feet quiet.
"Make your mouth quiet"	
"Make your hands quiet"	

Note that the instructions are all in the positive vein describing a desired behavior for the child to emit.

Another class of stimulus manipulation is modelling. Bandura (1969) and others have documented the modelling effects of children observing other children and learning from that observation, especially if the model is receiving reinforcement for specific behaviors. Putting a new child with another child or a group of children who already have learned and are demonstrating appropriate desired behaviors often facilitates the development of those behaviors.

Consequence Manipulation

Another way to manage behavior is to provide consequences for its occurrence (McReynolds, 1970). At least two procedures are available. If positive consequences (accelerators) follow the behavior, its frequency will be increased (accelerated). If negative consequences (decelerators) follow the behavior, its frequency will be decreased (decelerated). Money, smiling, saying "Good," and giving exchangeable tokens are generally thought of as positive events (accelerators). Ignoring, frowning, saying "No," and removing exchangeable tokens are generally viewed as negative events (decelerators).

The teacher seeks out positive or negative behaviors already in the repertoire of the child and provides appropriate positive or negative consequences. Even the most intractable child will demonstrate some positive behavior. This behavior should be positively reinforced and undesirable behavior ignored.

It is important to determine the valence of a particular consequence. Sometimes consequent events may appear initially to be clearly positive or negative, but only observation of their effects on the behavior will accurately determine their valence. Giving certain items to a child may turn out to be reinforcing only for the teacher. A simple, functional measure of the effectiveness of a reinforcer (accelerator) is to remove it and observe the resultant effect on the child's behavior. Observation of children's play and/or asking them or their parents about things they like will provide information about what is reinforcing to the children.

A token system has proved to be valuable in teaching. This system provides for the use of tokens (plastic chips, styrofoam stars, or beans) to be given the child immediately after each performance of a desirable behavior. These tokens are saved and later traded for a prize, or "back-up" reinforcer, such as a little toy or a piece of candy. There is little inherent value in the tokens themselves therefore they must be given value by being exchanged for items which are reinforcing. The tokens provide for a constant monitoring of the reinforcement process for both the child and the teacher. Some children may have to be taught the value of the tokens by having them explained or permitting them to be exchanged for back-up reinforcers several times during the first session. Eventually the child learns to save the tokens for an exchange day once a week. There are many variations on the token system (Allyon and Azrin, 1968). It has been our experience that a simple token economy has been very effective in providing for motivation during training.

Negative consequences (decelerators) are also defined by their effect on the child's behavior. People have commonly used ignoring the child, removal of a token, or standing the child in the corner (time out) as negative consequences.

The administration of a decelerator or accelerator is commonly accompanied by a verbal description of the behavior, for example, "Your feet are quiet, good." (The teacher also gives a token.) Or, "Your feet are noisy, you lose a token." (The teacher also removes a token.)

It is important to deliver the token and/or social reinforcer immediately after the desired response has been emitted. Of equal importance is the gradual reduction of the number of token reinforcers so that the behavior comes under the control of fewer token reinforcers and more social reinforcers. In the initial phases the teacher will administer many tokens, as the child's behavior improves the teacher can give fewer and fewer tokens and proportionately more social reinforcers. The teacher will come to expect longer and longer periods of desired behavior for which tokens or social approval can be administered. The effects of reinforcement schedules are shown below.

Schedule	Immediate Effect	Long Term Effect	When to Use
100%	good	poor	To establish a new behavior
50%	fair	fair	To maintain a behavior
10%	poor	good	To maintain a behavior over a long period of time

When the teacher is attempting to teach a new behavior or to increase a low frequency desired behavior, a 100 percent schedule should be used. As the child demonstrates more desired behavior, the schedule can be changed until only an occasional reinforcer

(10 percent) is given. This procedure has the effect of maintaining the behavior over long time periods. It also aids in transferring the behavior to those situations when the teacher is not present to give reinforcement. The effects of various schedules of reinforcement on behavior are well-documented (Ferster and Skinner, 1956; Bandura, 1969; Honig, 1966).

The same token economy is used in the language training program for accelerating language behavior. This system was discussed in Chapter Two. The reinforcement schedules for token administration are written into the programs.

A rule of thumb which the teacher may follow is to pick the least frequent desired behavior and focus on it until it increases in frequency. The reinforcement schedule on that behavior is eventually reduced. The teacher may then pick the next least frequent desired behavior and focus on it. This is continued until the child is sitting at his desk, ready, attending to the teacher, and responding when asked. Several samples of the total behavior management system are shown below.

Stimulus	Response	Consequences
teacher desk "Sit at your desk"	sits at desk	"Good, you are sitting at your desk" (Teacher gives a token).
teacher	looks at teacher	"Good, you are looking at me" (Teacher gives a token).
teacher	looks away	(Teacher ignores) or "You are looking away, you lose a token" (Teacher takes away a token).

The teacher should focus on positive behaviors in an attempt to increase them. This will also decrease their negative correlates (a child cannot look at the teacher and away at the same time).

Special Behaviors and Procedures

Some children with language problems will also exhibit bizarre, highly undesirable, negative behaviors. It is beyond the scope of this book to describe procedures for managing these children. The reader is referred to other sources such as Yates (1970); Ullman and Krasner (1965);

114

Sloane and MacAulay (1968); Ulrich, Stachnik, and Mabry (1966); and Eysenck (1964). The reader should also refer to articles from such journals as the *Journal of Applied Behavior Analysis* (Wolf, M., editor) and *Behaviour Research and Therapy* (Eysenck, H., editor). It is necessary to develop powerful strategies using both decelerators and accelerators to train certain children (autistic children, for example) to attend to the task of learning to talk.

One special behavior in the purview of this book which occurs occasionally in the conduction of the language programs themselves is "nonresponding." Children may not respond either because the program step is too hard or because of a behavior problem. Generally, nonresponding has been treated as a behavior problem. For the child who persists in nonresponding during a session on the language programs, the following procedure has proved helpful:

1. 1st time NR, go on with the program. (1st NR)
2. 2nd time NR, go on with the program. (2nd NR)
3. 3rd time NR say, "When you are ready to work raise your hand." (3rd NR)
4. If child raises hand and responds, go on with the program.
5. If child raises hand but doesn't respond, wait five minutes (4th NR)
6. After five minutes say, "Are you ready to work?"
7. If he says "Yes" and works, go on with the program.
8. If he says "No" or doesn't work, wait ten minutes. (5th NR)
9. After ten minutes say, "Are you ready to work?"
10. If he says "Yes" and works, go on with the program.
11. If he says "No" or doesn't work, wait until the end of language time.
12. If the child is still not working when language time is over, he misses the entire following activity and/or must make up the language training period during recess, juice and cookies, or some other play period.

This procedure is essentially a "time-out" process. It is time wasting if the teacher is working with only one child. If working with two or more children, the teacher can continue with the other child or children while the first one is waiting. If the activity which follows is not a particularly reinforcing one, missing it may have little effect.

Behavior management is essential to and an important part of the success of any teaching program. It is vital that the child attend to the learning task. This is the first goal of any teaching strategy and can usually be accomplished with positive means. It can and should be carried out concurrently with the language training.

SUPPORTIVE PERSONNEL AND EQUIPMENT

Teacher-Aides

The teacher administers the tests and language programs, and teacher-aides may be very helpful. These aides are often referred to as volunteers, auxillary members, paraprofessionals, or subprofessionals. They generally have little or no professional training. Aides in the language programs need only the qualifications of speaking adequate English themselves, interest in helping children, and time to work. They may be high school students, retired teachers, college students, housewives, etc. We have used a number of teacher-aides to help both in behavior management and in running the program. The aide training program to be described below was developed in the Children's House setting. Not all of it will be essential to aides' performance in other settings.

Aides first observe for one or two sessions. They are then given a copy of and asked to read Patterson and Gullion's (1968) *Living With Children*. The teacher discusses information from the book with them and answers their questions about it. The application of social learning principles to the teaching setting they have been observing is explained to them by the teacher.

A four-step process of teaching both behavior management and the language programs is used:

1. Explain   They are told what to look for and the situation is described.

2. Observe   They watch for specific activities and behavior.

3. Participate   They engage in the activity under the teacher's supervision.

4. Administer   They carry out the activity with minimal supervision from the teacher.

To teach the behavior management system, the aides receive a list of desired and undesired behaviors (see page III for a partial list) which they are to observe throughout a session or two. Next they are given the list of instructions (see page III for a partial list). They practice these under supervision. Finally, they are given tokens to dispense for desired behaviors along with the instructions. They dispense these throughout the session during language time and other activities. With these skills, aides can be extremely helpful to the teacher in managing the children.

Concurrent with training in behavior management, we train teacher-aides in the administration of programs and language activities. They are first given written information about the programs (actually a simplified version of this chapter and Chapter Two), and they then carry out language program activities. The sequence followed is shown below:

1. Scoring
2. Recording language for criterion tests
3. Recording language for show and tell
4. Charting
5. Giving a language program including scoring
6. Conducting show and tell time

Not all aides will learn all of these procedures. Much depends upon the time they are able to spend, their desire to learn more, and their basic ability. All aides have learned to score because it is a fairly straightforward task. They are told to keep score and indicate to the teacher when the child has attained criterion on a step. They score while the teacher carries out the language programs in the group setting. This permits the teacher to conduct a relatively large group. All aides have learned to record language during criterion tests and spontaneous language. The teacher will help them by repeating what the child has said if the child is relatively unintelligible and/or intelligible only to the teacher. Most aides have learned to chart and to administer a program step. They are taught the individual steps by the teacher each day until they have learned the code and can interpret it themselves. Some aides come only once a week, while others come daily. Those who come intermittently usually never progress beyond the one-step-in-a-program stage; those who come more often can eventually learn to run two or more children stimultaneously. Very few aides who come weekly learn to administer show and tell because this process is quite complicated. The show and tell period is a critical one during which previously learned language forms are evoked and reinforced and new language forms are tested.

Two problems are demonstrated by most aides, especially those who come infrequently. The first is speed of presentation: they are unable to work at the high rate of presentation usually employed by the teacher. The second is response evaluation. Although their evaluation of the children's language response is generally equal to the teacher's, as corroborated by informal reliability probes, they may have difficulty with a child whose articulation, semantic processing, or behavior is quite deviant. Occasionally the aides inadvertently reinforce incorrect responses which the teacher has to correct at a later time.

We have reported above on the conduct of aide training programs and the aides themselves. Most of our experience has been with intermittent aides, that is, those who come only once a week. They are easier to find in a practical sense, very available to any teacher in any community.

The other group of aides—those who spend more time in the program—generally perform very well and can learn to carry out the programs almost as well as the teacher. They usually learn to execute all of the activities short of testing and case selection. Their response evaluation and program administration are comparable to the teachers'.

Aides can be very helpful adjuncts to the language programs. Simply having them score testing can remove a large burden from the teacher who is trying to carry out language programs with a group of children. The teacher is encouraged to seek out aides and to train them to their capacity in intellect and time in order to assist the teacher in the conduction of the language programs.

The entire aide training program is available from the authors. However, with the information in Chapter Two and this chapter, one should be able to train aides to perform quite well in settings limited to language training.

Parents

As discussed earlier, parents are involved in the language training programs through the IHC or Initiate Home Carryover procedures. Language handicapped children frequently present behavior problems and parents express concern about them. In order to help the parents with their children's behavior problems at home, they participate in a training course in behavioral management using the book, *Living With Children* (Patterson and Gullion, 1968); another useful book is *Parents*

Are Teachers (Becker, 1971). The course helps the parents to cope effectively with the child's behavior at home and aids them in understanding the behavior principles employed in the language training periods. This training course has commonly run for five one-hour sessions and follows the outline given in Table II.

The parents are given information about behavior management much like that discussed here. They actually engage in modification activities and keep records (charts) of their children's progress in accelerating or decelerating certain behaviors. In some especially difficult cases, we have also gone into the home setting and worked with the parents there.

Occasionally parents have served as teacher aides, but we usually suggest that they work with children other than their own. It is possible that in the future we will develop and refine the language training activities to the point where the parent may be taught initially how to work with the child on language at home. More research is needed before this can be done.

Teaching Machines

It is theoretically possible to put the entire language teaching program on a teaching machine (Cram, 1961). This machine could be a tape recorder, a language master, a video tape recorder, or a more elaborate, com-

---

Table 11   Outline for Parent-Training Program*

Living With Children or Who Is Training Whom

Session I—Principles of Learning
> Reward (Types and Timing)
> Punishment
> Extinction

Session II—Behavior Targets
> Choosing Appropriate Targets
> Breaking Them Down into Bite Sizes
> Putting Them in Order

Session III—Measuring Success of Teacher (Parent)
> Measurement
> Record Keeping
> Improving Programs with Feedback

Session IV—Homework Assignments

Session V—Parents on Their Own as Behavior Modifiers

---

*Courtesy of Dr. Gene England, Director, Behavioral Sciences Institute

---

puterized teaching machine. The only human activity necessary is the judgment about the adequacy of the child's response. This must be done by another human being. We have tested both audio- and video-taped stimulus-model presentations and found them to be equally as effective as the "live" teacher. Counters and computers are available to handle the scoring and criterion processes leaving the teacher with only the task of pressing a "right" button for correct responses and a "wrong" button for incorrect responses.

We are presently developing a computer-aided language teaching machine. However, our present concern is with teaching the language program to teachers—and through them to the millions of children who need this type of language·training. We think language capability is likely to occur sooner through the use of live teachers and aides than it will through machines. Language training is still a most human effort (Bradfield, 1970).

Summary

In this chapter the teacher was presented with techniques and discussion concerning behavior management and ancillary language training activities related to the language programs themselves. The core elements in the language teaching process are the language programs themselves, but ancillary activities are vital to the appropriate delivery and measurement of said programs.

References

Ayllon, T. and Azrin, N. *The token economy: A motivational system for therapy and rehabilitation.* New York: Appleton-Century-Crofts, 1968.

Bandura, A. *Principles of behavior modification.* New York: Holt, Rinehart and Winston, Inc., 1969.

Bangs, T. Evaluating children with language delay. *Journal of Speech and Hearing Disorders*, 1961, *26*, 16-18.

Becker, W. *Parents are teachers.* Champaign, Ill.: Research Press, 1971.

Berry, M. *Language disorders of children: The bases and diagnoses.* New York: Appleton-Century-Crofts, 1969.

Bloom, L. *Language development: Form and function in emerging grammars.* Research monograph no. 59. Cambridge: M.I.T. Press, 1970.

Bradfield, R. (Ed.) *Behavior modification: The human effort.* San Rafael: Dimensions Publishing Co., 1970.

Carrow, M. The development of auditory comprehension of language structure in children. *Journal of Speech and Hearing Disorders,* 1968, *33,* 99-111.

Crabtree, M. *The Houston test for language development.* Houston: Houston Test Company, 1958.

Cram, D. *Explaining teaching machines and programming.* San Francisco: Fearon Publishers, 1961.

Dunn, L. *Peabody picture vocabulary test.* Minneapolis: American Guidance Service, 1959.

Englemann, S. *The basic concept inventory: Field research edition.* Chicago: Follett Educational Corporation, 1967.

Eysenck, H. (Ed.) *Experiments in behavior therapy.* New York: The MacMillan Co., 1964.

Ferster, C. and Skinner, B. *Schedules of reinforcement.* New York: Appleton-Century-Crofts, 1956.

Haring, N. and Lovitt, T. Operant methodology and educational technology in special education. In N. Haring and R. Schiefelbusch (Eds.), *Methods in special education.* New York: McGraw-Hill Book Company, 1967.

Haring, N. and Phillips, E. *Educating emotionally disturbed children.* New York: McGraw-Hill Book Company, 1962.

Hewett, F. *The emotionally disturbed child in the classroom.* Boston: Allyn and Bacon, Inc., 1968.

Honig, W. (Ed.) *Operant behavior: Areas of research and application.* New York: Appleton-Century-Crofts, 1966.

Johnson, D. and Myklebust, H. *Learning disabilities.* New York: Grune and Stratton, 1967.

Johnson, W., Darley, F., and Spriestersbach, D. *Diagnostic methods in speech pathology.* New York: Harper and Row, 1963.

Kirk, S., McCarthy, J., and Kirk, W. *The Illinois test—Psycholinguistic abilities,* rev. ed. Urbana: University of Illinois Press, 1968.

Lee, L. Developmental sentence types: A method for comparing normal and deviant syntactical development. *Journal of Speech and Hearing Disorders,* 1966, *31,* 311-330.

Lee, L. *The Northwestern syntax screening test.* Evanston, Illinois: Northwestern University Press, 1969.

Lee, L. A screening test for syntax development. *Journal of Speech and Hearing Disorders,* 1970, *35,* 103-112.

Lee, L. and Canter, S. Developmental sentence scoring: A method for measuring syntactic development in children's spontaneous speech. *Journal of Speech and Hearing Disorders,* 1971, *36,* 315-340.

Lillywhite, H., Bradley, D., Nelson, D., Holeman, L., Nicon, J., and Fletcher, S. Oregon language profile. Personal communication, 1970.

McReynolds, L. Contingencies and consequences in speech therapy. *Journal of Speech and Hearing Disorders,* 1970, *35,* 12-24.

Mecham, M., Jex, J., and Jones, J. *Utah test of language development,* rev. ed. Salt Lake City: Communication Research Associates, 1967.

Menyuk, P. *Sentences children use.* Cambridge: M.I.T. Press, 1969.

Miner, L. Scoring procedures for the length-complexity index: A preliminary report. *Journal of Communication Disorders,* 1969, *2,* 224-240.

Muma, J. Hypothesis testing: Ten techniques to facilitate language learning. *Acta Symbolica,* 1970, *1,* 43-46.

Patterson, G. and Gullion, E. *Living with children.* Champaign, Ill.: Research Press, 1968.

Shriner, T. A comparison of selected measures with psychological scale values and language development. *Journal of Speech and Hearing Research,* 1967, *10,* 828-835.

Shriner, T. A review of mean length of response as a measure of expressive language development in children. *Journal of Speech and Hearing Disorders,* 1969, *34,* 61-68.

Skinner, B. *Science and human behavior.* New York: The MacMillan Company, 1953.

Sloane, H. and MacAulay, B. (Eds.) *Operant procedures in remedial speech and language training.* Boston: Houghton-Mifflin Co., 1968.

Terman, L. and Merrill, M. *Stanford-Binet intelligence scale: Manual for the third revision, form L-M.* Boston: Houghton-Mifflin Co., 1960.

Ullman, L. and Krasner, L. (Eds.) *Case studies in behavior modification.* New York: Holt, Rinehart and Winston, 1965.

Ulrich, R., Stachnik, T., and Mabry, T. (Eds.) *Control of human behavior.* Glenview, III.: Scott, Foresman and Co., 1966.

Walker, H., Mattson, R., and Buckley, N. Special class placement as a treatment alternative for deviant behavior in children. In F. Benson (Ed.), *Modifying deviant social behaviors in classroom settings.* Eugene, Ore.: University of Oregon Press, 1969.

Weschler, D. *Weschler intelligence scale for children.* New York: The Psychological Corporation, 1949.

Yates, A. *Behavior therapy.* New York: John Wiley and Sons, 1970.

Zimmerman, I., Steiner, V., and Evatt, R. *Preschool language manual.* Columbus, Ohio: Charles E. Merrill Publishing Co., 1969.

4 Accountability

Obligations

Anyone who presumes to put forth a suggested plan of instructional strategy takes on certain obligations. The most pressing of these is to provide evidence for the validity of the procedure. That evidence should be sufficiently adequate to permit the reader to make judgments about the strengths and weaknesses of the procedure.

Teachers who read such material sometimes become impatient with results, preferring to move straight on to the actual clinical activity; however, they, too, have a serious obligation. They should understand what a particular program will do with children who are to be placed in it. Thus, both author and reader have obligations which relate to the data. Both parties must uphold those obligations for the welfare of the prospective student.

The main point of the matter is that inspection of the data should permit the teacher to determine if the past history of the procedure justifies using it in a test probe. The cost of such a study can be expensive. First, the teacher must become proficient in the execution of the procedure if it is to have a valid trial. Secondly, the children who are used in the test, by definition, are being excluded from other possible procedures which may benefit them. Therefore, it is very important that the reported success of the program be of sufficient magnitude and credibility to justify the probe.

The process which a teacher should use in deciding upon a procedure basically involves three questions. Is the intended application of the procedure appropriate? Should I try it? Should I use it routinely? Obviously the first question should be whether or not the procedure is designed for the type of situation where its use is being considered. The misuse, or more appropriately, misapplication of procedures has resulted in far too much failure for teachers and students alike. But, if a teacher can carefully examine a procedure, it is usually possible to determine whether that procedure is appropriate for the population and the behavioral objective that is desired. If this can be successfully determined, the second question can be asked.

The answer as to whether or not to try a procedure as an exploratory test probe involves data that are reported for that procedure as a part of the validation. This typically involves before and after measures on some type of criterion test or other objective measures of performance. There are two primary objectives with which this type of information is meant to deal. The first is the documentation of evidence of a meaningful change in the target performance in question. The data should show not only a credible amount of change, but also they should demonstrate that the direction of that change was both consistent from subject to subject as well as predictable for each subject. The second objective of this type of data is to demonstrate that the observed changes in the test measures can, with reasonable assurance, be attributed to the procedure rather than to the research design or some spurious artifact. These two aspects of the data are called reliability and validity (Sidman, 1960).

In order to properly evaluate the probe once it has been started, the teacher must keep track of the results that the procedure is generating. The first information which must be obtained and evaluated is the run data. Run data refer to the operating characteristics of the program. This includes information on response accuracy, number of responses necessary to complete the program, and number of instructional hours needed to complete the program. This information permits the teacher to compare the running characteristics of the test probe with the running characteristics reported for the procedure generally. It then can be determined whether or not the test probe was executed in a satisfactory manner. If it was satisfactory, then the target performance can be evaluated.

The second type of information which must be obtained is the before and after criterion test performance data. Out of casual interest these data can be compared to the original results given for the procedure. However, the most important decision concerns whether the test probe results are good enough in and of themselves to justify the continued, if not expanded, use of the procedure. The original validation data can only aid in answering the first two questions—particularly the second. It has little actual bearing on the final decision to fully incorporate a program into the teaching scheme.

If the first two questions are satisfactorily answered, the last question can be considered. The decision to use a program in the standard routine of the instructional scheme demands that the data from the test probe be highly positive. In any final sense a procedure is justifiable only when it works for that teacher in that setting and if the instructional environment can reasonably be expected to support the use of the procedure.

Throughout the first portions of this book we have tried to provide information relating to the first question about appropriateness. Presuming that the reader would not reach this point if programmed conditioning for language were totally inappropriate, we will try to provide validation and information about the second question—Should I try it?

Protocol

A description of our experience with programmed conditioning for language is as follows. Seventy thousand hours of programming experience and over 1.5 million responses have been accumulated. These figures represent many different situations and many different teachers and types of children. The "prime" testing sample was a day school for nonlanguage, preschool children called Children's House. That school was staffed by one full-time teacher and volunteer aides. There was one three-hour class of seven children in the morning and seven other children in the three-hour afternoon class.

During each class, programmed conditioning sessions covered 90 minutes. The remainder of the time was used for less formal language situations such as juice and cookies, recess, and show and tell time. The programming was carried out during two 45-minute sessions. The first session usually included the entire class. The second session was frequently broken up into smaller groups of two and three children.

We endeavored to keep this particular subject population as reasonably homogeneous as possible. We tried to obtain preschool children who had normal intellectual potential but who were not talking. These children were often quite hyperactive—that is, they could sit at a desk for no longer than twelve seconds. These children were frequently labled dysphasic. Other classifications of children, such as mentally retarded, autistic, hard of hearing, delayed language, non-English speaking, etc., also were run on the programs in different settings.

The prime test population, Children's House, represents our longest and most consistent language programming experience. The major portion of the data is from that population. However, we will report results from other classifications as well.

The overall protocol for language assessment for the

Children's House population included the following items. An original diagnostic test battery comprised of the Illinois Test of Psycholinguistic Abilities (Kirk, McCarthy, and Kirk, 1968); the Northwestern Syntax Screening Test (Lee, 1970); the Peabody Picture Vocabulary Test (Dunn, 1959); selected items from the Stanford-Binet (Terman and Merrill, 1960); Weschler (Weschler, 1949); and the Goodenough Draw A Person Test (Goodenough, 1926) were used. This test battery was administered by the diagnostic team of the clinical services department of the Behavioral Sciences Institute (formerly the Monterey Institute for Speech and Hearing). This procedure was used to determine the need for language training and was not especially considered to be part of the programmed protocol. All children seen at the Institute were put through this type of omnibus evaluation. If it was determined that language training was needed, a more specific diagnostic procedure was used.

The Programmed Conditioning Language Test (PCLT), which is a sentence repetition test, was used to determine which of the programs in the curriculum were needed. Next, a criterion test was given before and after each program was administered. That test consisted of items equivalent to the last steps in the target program. A placement system was used to determine where in each program a child should start. Three conversational situations were then monitored to obtain samples of conversational language. These last samples were taken regularly through the entire period. Conversational samples were evaluated in terms of percent correct responding. A transcript of the children's language was analyzed for correct usage of certain specified linguistic targets. The actual number of correct usages divided by the total possible correct usages multiplied by 100 equals the percent correct responding. This last measure in addition to the Northwestern Syntax Screening Test (NSST) and the PCLT were the measures which were taken most frequently on the Children's House population. Also, they are the measures which we will use most frequently to report our results.

Other samples of nonlanguage children who were not placed in the prime testing situation because of other characteristics (such as hearing loss, mental retardation, autism, etc.) were placed in other clinical environments at the Institute. The same basic protocol and the same language programs were run on these children. Also, there were a number of language programming situations which were run by trained teachers who were working in other locations and who were not members of the Institute's staff. The testing protocol for these situations varied from that reported for the Children's House and Institute populations. Each of these special situations will be described later.

Children's House—The Prime Sample

The decision to keep the Children's House population as close to the label of dysphasic as possible was because of certain characteristics of this group of children. Basically, dysphasic children are very active, normally intelligent children who may have organic brain damage and who do not talk. They have no gross overriding characteristics such as hearing loss, cerebral palsy, or mental retardation. They will be enrolled in the public school system and will experience severe difficulty before or during their first grade because of the language problem. They are prime candidates for special education. However, with normal language usage these children will suffer only the normal perils of public education along with their classmates. Dysphasic children are very frequently encountered by language teachers in special classes because their lack of any remarkable handicap (other than their not talking) usually gets them placed initially in a regular class. From there they are referred to the special teacher.

Our reasoning was that if a language training procedure could be designed for children who were on the borderline between success and failure in our educational system, with only minor topographical alterations it might be successfully applied to those children with language problems of both a more serious and of a less serious nature. It is important to remember that the goal was and is to teach language to children. . .any children. It is *language* that is being taught, not different kinds of etiologies.

The following data were obtained over a four-year period. The average entering age of the 43 children in the Children's House population was 4.7 years, ranging from 3 to 7 years. The ratio of boys to girls was twenty to one. Generally speaking, the number of boys having language problems is usually reported to be higher than the number of girls; however, the imbalance is not as great as that reported here. We could find no special reason for such a heavy imbalance in this particular instance.

The mean receptive and expressive ability for these children prior to programming was below the tenth percentile for children their age as measured by the NSST. On the PCLT the mode score for the test sample was nine percent correct while the mode score for normal children of that age was 100 percent. Figure 26 shows the distribution of receptive and expressive NSST scores for 18 incoming children. Although the NSST is not a statistically normalized test, it does give some general information about the ability of the children. The NSST is meant to be a screening test, and its results should be viewed only as a general statement rather than as a highly discrete discription; however, it does provide two important pieces of information. First, it is clear that the test population is obviously performing below the norms on this test at all ages reported. Second, it provides confirmation of similar results obtained on the PCLT which is specific to the language curriculum.

Figure 26   Distribution of Receptive and Expressive NSST Scores by Age for 18 Incoming Nonlanguage Children. The numbers 90, 50, and 10 Refer to the Respective Percentile Distributions Reported for Normal Language Children.

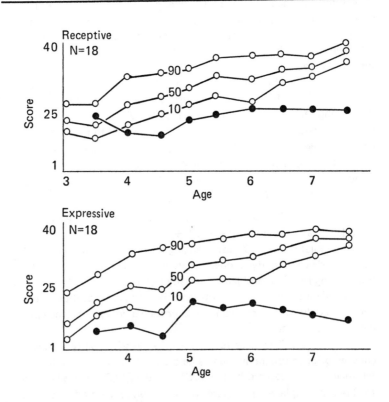

There is an important difference between the NSST and the PCLT. The NSST is a screening test instrument which is designed to describe the progress of normal language development. On the other hand, the PCLT is a screening test which is specifically designed to yield information about which programs in the available curriculum are needed for a given child. With the PCLT, there is no intent to define normal language acquisition or performance. Despite this difference, the results of both these tests strongly indicate a very marginal language performance by the test population. The typical verbal behavior of these children included some naming responses and occasionally some jargon behavior. It was not unusual to find children who did not demonstrate even this much language performance.

A high rate of physical activity and distractability was noted to occur in about 60 percent of the children. This necessitated the use of the behavioral management procedures which were discussed in Chapter Three. No child was started on language programming until the hyperactivity and distractability were reduced to a manageable level.

One further note of explanation is needed prior to discussing the results of our language work with these children. It was mentioned earlier that the data were collected over a four-year period on a total of 43 children. At any one time no more than 14 children were enrolled (seven in each class). Some children completed the program curriculum before others and new children took their place. Thus, there was a constant mix of "old" and "new" children in the program. The situation made data collection somewhat complex; therefore, we tended to ask specific questions—either during discrete time periods or about specific children. Questions on, before, and after criterion test scores for particular programs might be pursued for a period of six months. Then, new and different measures might be obtained on other aspects of the program. To try to ask all the questions about all of the children in all of the lessons would have completely overwhelmed our data retrieval and analysis system. Only the program run data, which will be presented later, include data on all of the subjects. The result of this was that each report may be based upon a different number of subjects. The number of subjects reported for any one result is merely the function of how many children happened to be enrolled or were being monitored at the time that particular information was gathered.

Generally, the determination of the correctness of a response has been a relatively simple activity when the rules for response evaluation, outlined in Chapters Two and Three, were followed. To support this observation, a reliability probe with the teacher and an independent observer was conducted for children on different steps in different programs in both group and individual settings. The mean percentage of agreement between the teacher and an independent observer in the individual settings was 100 percent, while in the group setting it was 97.1 percent.

Student Performance

During the four-year test sample the students accumulated a total of 30,240 student class hours. Of this amount, they spent 20,160 total student hours in language programming and language related activities. The actual amount of program run time was 2,160 hours. The total number of responses recorded for all students at Children's House was 288,000.

The mean accuracy with which the students responded on the programs was 89.9 percent with σ = 16.1. The mean number of responses needed to complete an entire program was 794 with σ = 102. The mean time needed to complete an entire program was 3.7 hours in the group situation. The earlier programs in the curriculum tended to have a lower accuracy and a longer run time than did later programs. Part of this was probably due to the fact that on the first few programs the child was having to learn the protocol of the lesson as well as the correct response. Also, the more language a child had, the easier it was for him to pick up new language. In addition, if there were any vestiges of behavior problems they would be operating during the early programs.

The "Naming Nouns" (No. 2) program typically ran about 20 percentage points lower than the mean accuracy for all programs. The accuracy score tended to go up from that point until the "Is" (No. 4) or "Is Verbing" (No. 5) programs, at which time the accuracy leveled off at the low to mid 90s. Figure 27 is a pooled data performance chart for ten children on the "What Is" program (No. 7). The configuration and characteristics of the response accuracy line of this chart are typical of performance charts on programmed conditioning. The histogram at the far right of the graph indicates the difference in pre- and post-criterion test measures for this group of ten children. Both the accuracy level of the chart and the pre- and post-measures agree favorably with similar data on other programs which have been presented elsewhere (Gray and Fygetakis, 1968a and b; Gray, 1970; Fygetakis and Gray, 1970).

Figure 27 does give information about how students performed on the "What Is" (No. 7) program. However, it also has been noted that performance improves as a child goes further along through the curriculum. Figure 28 shows the change in the average accuracy of performance on the pre- and post-criterion measures for any one child on any one program. Students go into a program with an average

Figure 27   **Mean Data Performance Chart for 10 Children on the *What Is Interrogative* Program. Histogram At Far Right Indicates the Pre- and Post-Criterion Test Measures**

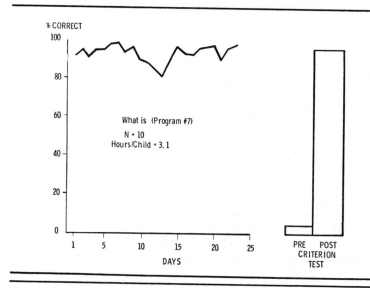

Figure 28   **Mean Pre- and Post-Criterion Test Performance for Any One Child On Any One Program**

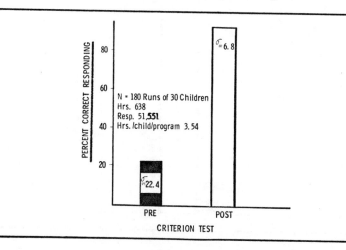

accuracy of 22 percent and complete the program with an average accuracy of 93 percent. This 71 percentage point gain is substantial even though it is less than that for the "What Is" (No. 7) program alone.

The entering score of 22 percent may appear to be rather high considering the fact that these children have been found to have little, if any, language behavior. The reason for such a high entering score is that as a child goes through more programs he begins to acquire some marginal ability on other, not yet taught, forms. This is to be expected if the child is, in fact, gaining language ability as he goes along.

The criterion test is very close to the actual programming experience. Thus, a possibly more encompassing type of pre- and post-measurement of the language performance of the children would be the PCLT. This brief test also is tied to the programs, but since it scans the entire curriculum and is not limited to the most recent program, as is the criterion test, it does tend to have more perspective. Figure 29 presents the PCLT test results compared at a one-year interval for ten children. The increase in response accuracy over this time interval is 55 percentage points. The 61 hours of programming per child represents the first 61 hours of training. Thus the post score of

Figure 29   Mean PCLT Test Results Compared At a One-Year Interval for 10 Children

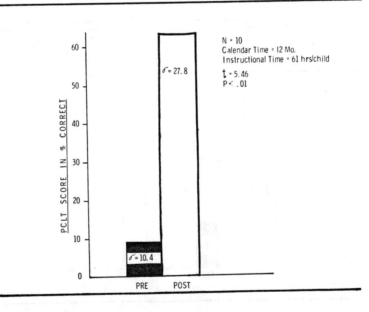

N = 10
Calendar Time = 12 Mo.
Instructional Time = 61 hrs/child
t = 5.46
P < .01

$\sigma = 27.8$

$\sigma = 10.4$

64 percent is not a terminal score but merely the score that was achieved one calendar year (or 61 programming hours) after the pre-score. The difference between the pre- and post-test scores is significant beyond the p=.01 level (t=5.46/df=9).

It can be concluded that there was some type of increment in language performance; whether that change is due to the passage of time and maturation or to the programming per se has not been established. The usual method for ascertaining this fact is to simultaneously run a control group. However, this becomes a very complex issue in the present situation. A control group for this population must, by definition, be preschool children with normal intellectual potential who don't talk. Since the dysphasic child has a history of nonlanguage performance, it is unlikely that he will spontaneously begin to talk in the one-year period prior to school. Thus, to put him in a control group where he is purposely excluded from any special type of language training program is, in most cases, to sentence him to educational failure in school. Since language training quite frequently can make the difference between failure and success, the decision to exclude becomes very consequential. The ethical and moral persuasions of this issue are grave and vigorously argue against this type of test.

There is another resolution to the problem. It is possible to compare the rate of growth of language between normal language children and the sample population. While 14 children from the sample population with a mean age of 5.0 years were on programming, two different NSST measures were taken. Seven months separated the two measures. The change in NSST scores over this period was compared to the change reported for normal children on the norms of the NSST for a six-month period. There were no mean regression effects found in the data: figure 4.0 points expressively and a change of 4.5 points receptively. Normal language five-year-olds gained approximately 1.0 point both expressively and receptively. Although they are operating at two quite different levels of language proficiency, the program children were showing an improvement in language ability that was four times as great as normals.

Receptive Vs. Expressive Performance

Of additional interest in Figure 30 is the observation that the apparent effect of an expressive-production curriculum of programs is distributed over receptive as well as expressive test measures. This argues against the position that nonverbal language performance must be trained prior to embarking upon a verbal production activity. This is not to deny that some "receptive" skills are imbedded in the programming activity. Rather, it is to point up the fact that all of the programs, with the exception of No. 1 (Identification of Nouns), require only verbal performance. More will be said about the meaning of this finding in terms of popular philosophy about language in Chapter Five.

Figure 30	Mean Change in NSST Scores Over Calendar Months Plotted for 14 Language Program Children

and for the Normative NSST Test Population. The Letters E and R Refer to Expressive and Receptive Scores

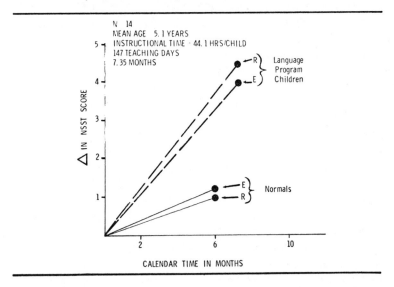

Support for the findings presented in Figure 30 are found in a somewhat similar observation about a different set of data presented in Figure 31. The bar (I) on the left group of histograms indicates the tested receptive ability of six children prior to programming. The center bar (1st) indicates the average receptive test scores for two of the six children when they were graduated directly into first grade. The right-hand bar (K) indicates the same information for the remaining four children who were graduated into kindergarten. The second set of histograms gives the same information about the tested expressive ability of the children. There is a noticeable change in both receptive and expressive test scores. It can be seen that there was a large difference between receptive and expressive test scores initially. It also would appear from the chart that there was a proportionately greater acceleration for expressive ability than for receptive ability, although in an absolute sense expression remains lower than reception. These data high-

Figure 31   Average NSST Scores for Six Children as a
               Function of Training on 13 Programs. In Both
               Groups of Histograms, the Left Hand Bar Which is
Identified With the Letter I Represents the Mean Receptive and
Expressive Scores for the Group of Six. The Center Bar of Both
Sets Which is Identified With the Symbol 1st Represents The Mean
Exiting Score for Two of the Children Who Went Into First Grade.
The Right-hand Histogram, Which is Identified With the Symbol K,
Represents the Mean Exiting Score for the Remaining Four Children
Who Were Transferred Directly into Kindergarten.

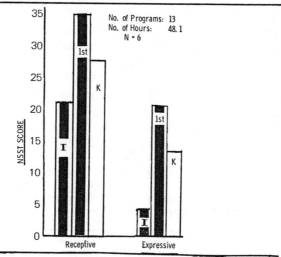

light a general statement about the effects of the programming on
tested receptive and expressive performance, i.e., that the programming
results in gains in both receptive and expressive ability with proportionately greater gains in expressive performance.

A different analysis of the data tends to confirm these
observations. When the change in expressive scores on the NSST is
plotted against the change in receptive scores for the sample population
as in Figure 32, it can be seen that (1) initially reception is greater than
expression and (2) for every unit increase in expression there is a cor-
respondingly smaller increase in reception. On the other hand, for the
normals the initial difference between reception and expression—while in
the same direction—is not as large as it was for the sample population.
Also, there is nearly a one to one correspondence between change in
expression and reception. Although the normals are at a higher level of
reception and expression test scores than the program sample, the children in the language programs are increasing their test performance at a
much greater rate, i.e., they are catching up.

Transfer of Training

In the Introduction, the concept of a mini-language was put forth. This discussion centered around the fact that if programmed conditioning were to be successful and practical, the student would have to be able to learn new rules on his own without having to be specifically taught every existing rule. This is known as transfer of training. If we now turn our attention to the question of training, we can see some of the effects of the programming. The term transfer of training here is taken to mean the increase in percent correct responding of a specific linguistic form as a function of going through preceding adjacent programs. That is, how much will the usage of an "Is Verbing" (No. 5) construction increase in accuracy as a function of the child having been on the "Is" (No. 4) program which immediately precedes it? In Figure 33 it can be seen that prior to programming for "Is" (No. 4) the accuracy of "Is" (No. 4) and "Is Verbing" (No. 5) constructions in conversational samples was zero. After programming for "Is" (No. 4) the accuracy for "Is" (No. 4) increased to 97 percent correct and the accuracy for "Is Verbing" (No. 5) increased to 20 percent for this child.

Figure 32 **The Change in NSST Expressive Scores Plotted as a Function of the Change in NSST Receptive Scores for Both the Sample Population (PC) and the NSST Normative Test Sample**

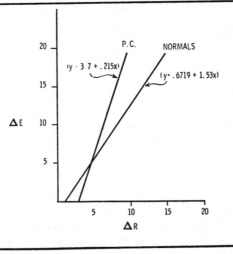

A more extended analysis of this same phenomenon can be seen in Figure 34. Here the accuracy for "What Is" (No. 7) in

Figure 33   Percent Correct Responses During Spontaneous Language Samples for One Child Taken Before and After Programmed Conditioning for *is*. Measurements were Taken for Is Constructions and Also For *Is Verbing* Constructions. (Gray and Fygetakis, 1968b.)

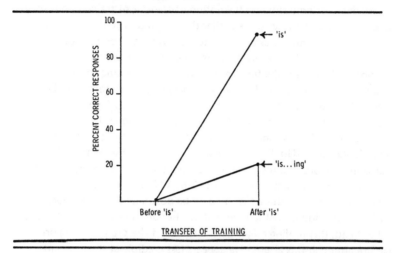

TRANSFER OF TRAINING

Figure 34   Mean Percent Correct Responses for Two Groups of Children on the *What Is* Construction. Measurements Were Taken During Spontaneous Language Samples Obtained at Four Different Time Periods in the Sequence of Programmed Conditioning Procedures. (Gray and Fygetakis, 1968b.)

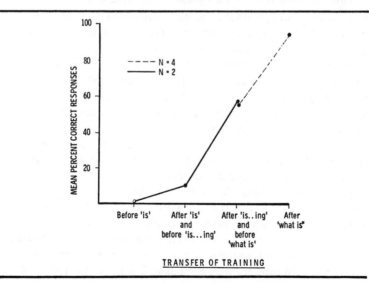

TRANSFER OF TRAINING

139

conversation is plotted as a function of going through the three program sequence of "Is" (No. 4), "Is Verbing" (No. 5), and "What Is" (No. 7). To confirm the third data point after "Is Verbing" (No. 5) and before "What Is" (No. 7), two different groups of children were plotted. These data not only support the notion of transfer of training, but they also are complimentary to the earlier discussion of a gradual increase in precriterion test measures as a function of programs completed.

One interesting observation which we have made and cannot explain yet is the finding that transfer of training (or nonprogrammed transformational growth) appears to observe some family class restrictions. That is, although the effect noted in Figure 34 is quite marked, there appears to be no effect upon other, less similar constructions. For instance, the two program sequence of "Is" (No. 4) and "Is Verbing" (No. 5), while dramatically affecting "What Is" (No. 7) performance, did nothing at all for performance on "He, She, and It" (No. 9) or other dissimilar programs such as "Singular and Plural Past Tense" (No. 23). At this point it could be postulated that there are various transformational families with rather discrete class lines. On the other hand, this finding might be an artifact of the programming procedure although this alternative appears less credible at the moment. Resolution of this problem must await further data.

Carryover

The term carryover is used in the present context to mean the ability of a child to use a newly learned linguistic construction in environments other than the language programming session. Typically, when a child is two-thirds of the way through a program we will begin to observe this use of the construction in areas less similar to the language programming session. His progression is as follows: show and tell, juice and cookies, playground, home, and finally school. Interestingly, the progression conforms generally to the geographic distance from the language programming class setting.

Language samples of five children (who were at varying levels in the programs) were selected from the show and tell periods for analysis. These samples were collected monthly over an eight-month period (September through April). A reliability probe, which included six different pairs of observers and five different children, revealed an average 81.5 percent agreement on the occurrence of specific words. The responses of the children were divided into words, phrases, and sentences. The percentages of the total number of responses emitted by each child in each category were computed. The percentages of words, phrases, and sentences for only the first (September) and the last (April) of the eight samples are shown in Figure 35.

Figure 35   **Mean Percent of Words, Phrases, and Sentences for Five Children During Show and Tell Time for Two Sampling Periods, I (September) II (April)**

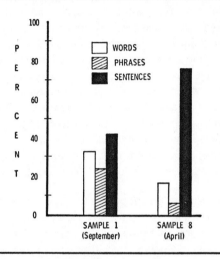

       During the first sample the children were using almost as many single word or phrase utterances as they were sentences. Only three of the five children did demonstrate sentences in the first sample. Eight months later in sample two, all of the children were using proportionately many more (76 percent) sentences. An analysis of the sentences revealed that 89.2 percent of them were correct. This compares favorably with the 89.9 percent accuracy, which the children demonstrated on the training programs. These data indicate that the children had learned to speak in sentences and had carried over this ability with a high degree of accuracy to the more spontaneous show and tell period.

       During the last four years that this project has been running, we have yet to observe the relapse of language performance after it had been established in the home setting via the carryover procedure. Although at first it might seem to be an extraordinary statement to make, the idea of no relapse of language should not be that unusual. Once learned, language performance becomes a universally used and reinforced skill. The environment is usually totally supportive of language performance. In fact, we doubt if it is possible to extinguish language from a person who has acquired it. It undoubtedly would be possible to extinguish the use of the verbal performance itself. But to extinguish or to cause the disappearance of the language skill and rules acquired by a person may be an entirely different matter.

To pursue further the issue of general language behavior, ten of the children who were in training were recorded on tape during their home activities (Ryan and Gray, 1971). A staff member who was not familiar to the child and who was not associated with the school or the school teacher went into the home for a one to two hour period. While there, she would attach a wireless microphone to the child. She then would sit in some inconspicuous place and, by means of an FM radio tape-recorder-receiver, recorded all the language of the child and those persons who talked to him. During this home sample probe a total of 20 hours of language behavior was recorded. The tapes were then returned to the Communications Laboratory of the Institute for analysis. All of the tapes were transcribed into longhand for detailed analysis. Inter-transcriber reliability for individual word recognition was 75 percent agreement and inter-transcriber reliability was 94.7 percent agreement.

Any attempt on our part to follow the child around and record or transcribe his utterances would have changed the normal environment to such a degree that it was not even attempted. Therefore, the use of a small wireless microphone permitted us to obtain a sample of language performance in a reasonably unobtrusive manner. The children did not demonstrate any preoccupation with or concern over wearing the microphone other than normal curiosity when it was first pinned on their clothing. Thus, our evaluation was that the validity of the sample was sufficiently high to warrant its acceptance as a representative sample.

There are five general observations concerning the language samples which are germane to this discussion. First, the most obvious characteristic was that the language performance was holding up in the home environment and was being used.

Second, one of the most important findings was that the home language performance samples showed that the children were using a much greater range of vocabulary and language construction at home than they did in the class setting at school. The transcriptions of show and tell language performance demonstrated a high usage of language forms that were taught on the programs with some occasional novel forms. The home samples, on the other hand, contained usages that could not be accounted for by specific language programming or program form transformational families.

The explanation for this disparity probably lies in the fact that the school environment—even the more social activities like show and tell—was arranged to provide us with a check on usage of programmed language forms. This prestructuring no doubt limited the range of utterances that the child used. The finding is a very important and critical one. Originally we indicated that if this method were to be successful, the language performance must begin to expand and develop without specific conditioning, otherwise the task would be too enormous to even attempt. This current finding, in conjunction with other findings about transfer of training, indicates that the mini-language concept does appear to be successful.

This knowledge of transfer of training and generalization in the natural environment also confirms the utility of the carryover procedure that is used at the end of each program. Although the procedure is rather simple and not very long, it appears to be sufficient to gain the desired behavior change.

Since the child was wearing the microphone, it was possible to record dialogues between him and his parents—usually his mother. The next three findings taken from the transcripts refer to these parent-child verbal interactions.

The third general finding is that parents tend to indiscriminately reinforce all verbal utterances made by the child. The fourth finding is that parents appear to understand nearly all utterances made by the child, even jargon utterances. And finally, parents did not do any correcting of error utterances nor did they engage in any activity that was identifiable as teaching.

In order to obtain some information about the possibility of differences between the parent-child dialogues of nonlanguage and normal language children, we initiated a small probe. We selected normal speaking children aged 3, 4, 5, and 6 years. After obtaining permission from the parents, we entered the home in a manner similar to that described for the language program children. Tape recordings were made of the conversations between child and parent just as they had been made for the other children.

From the data on these four children, three things were noted. First, the parents appeared to understand most of what the child said. This finding is similar to that reported for parents of nonlanguage children. Second, parents of normal language children would correct error responses of the child. This was done most typically by presenting a corrected model of the child's utterance. This was in contrast to the behavior of parents of nonlanguage children who evidenced little or no correcting behavior. Third, the parents of normal language children did not appear to reinforce error responses of the child. This, too, was in contrast to the behavior of parents of nonlanguage children who appeared to indiscriminately reinforce all utterances.

It should be remembered that these latter findings were only peripheral to the main purpose of this sampling project. Other than as statements of what occurred, these findings should not be used as the basis for substantial speculation concerning the reasons for the lack of language development originally, nor for differences between the language contingent behavior of parents of normal language and nonlanguage children.

The home language samples of the four normal children were also compared to those of the language program children. Only sentences were analyzed. The percentage of occurrence of various grammatical forms and the percentage of correct sentences were computed. These data are shown in Table 12.

Table 12   Mean Percentages of Grammatical Forms and Correct Sentences From the Home Setting for a Group (N 10) of Linguistically Divergent Children Who Were in Language Training and a Group of Normal Language Children (N 4)

| | Language Divergent | | Normal | | |
	Mean	S. D.	Mean	S. D.	t
Age	5.12	.99	5.1	1.1	.03
% Correct Sentences	61.69	19.40	86.80	8.76	2.30*
% Grammatical Forms					
Nouns	15.20	5.27	15.66	4.34	.14
Adjectives	2.30	1.59	3.33	2.42	.86
Adverbs	7.21	2.54	8.14	2.79	.56
Prepositions	3.62	3.51	4.01	1.14	.20
Possessives	2.82	2.38	2.70	1.88	.08
Indefinite Pronouns	8.95	4.95	9.62	2.69	.24
Personal Pronouns	23.17	4.40	19.91	2.57	1.28
Primary Verbs	23.51	4.98	20.62	4.46	.93
Secondary Verbs	3.96	2.69	2.87	.98	.73
Negatives	2.41	1.83	2.68	1.00	.26
Conjunctions	.54	.61	2.66	1.49	3.49*
Interrogative Reversals	2.62	2.47	5.13	3.13	1.46
WH Questions	3.64	2.91	2.59	3.59	.53

* p @ .05=t of 2.17 with df = 12.

Although the language divergent children were at various stages in the language training and in levels of language proficiency, as a group they demonstrated the use of all measured language forms. This finding supports the previous discussion on the use of language in the home setting by the language divergent children.

Because the sample of normal children was limited, the comparison between them and the language divergent children must be viewed only as a simple probe. In this comparison, the language divergent children were significantly different from the normals in only two aspects: they were less accurate in their sentence productions (61 percent vs. 86.80 percent) and they used fewer conjunctions (.54 percent vs. 2.66 percent). The difference in percentage correct for sentence usage is expected due to the fact that the children were still in training. The difference between the groups in the use of the conjunction was probably due to the fact that none of the children had been on the "Conjunction, and" program (No. 33).

Lest it appear that these language divergent children had normal language, it should be noted that a detailed, in-depth analysis of the subclasses of the general grammatical forms revealed that the normal language children used qualitatively more complex and sophisticated constructions than did the language-trained children (Ryan and Gray, 1971).

To summarize our experience with the prime population (Children's House) we may conclude that: (1) the language programs ran efficiently and resulted in target acquisition, (2) the children demonstrated transfer of training from one form to another, and (3) generalization of language was evidenced in the home setting.

Autistic Children. Although the term autistic does not have a highly specific behavioral definition, these children do have certain identifiable language characteristics in common. In terms of language performance, they fall into one of three very general categories. One group of autistic children will show virtually no verbal language performance. The extent of vocal communication, if present at all, is usually made up of a very few noises. These noises may or may not be accompanied by nonvocal gestures. It is not unusual to encounter tenacious clinical debates over whether to label such a child as autistic or receptively aphasic. According to our philosophy, it makes little difference what you call the child unless that decision has some strategic meaning for the training procedure. Since in our case it does not, we have arbitrarily elected to include all such performance examples under one heading for ease of discussion.

The second category includes children whose prosody and melody of verbal performance is reminiscent of the English inflectional pattern. However, the content of the performance is jargon. The output appears to be devoid of normal sounding words. The production effort on the part of the child is frequently quite animated and enthusiastic.

The third general category of language functioning is one in which the child demonstrates a highly developed grammar; however, the usage or content is frequently totally irrelevant to the situation. This child may talk normally for a brief period and then suddenly change the total content of the utterance to the point where it has no meaning to the listener whatsoever. Echolalia also may be present.

It should be emphasized that we are merely trying to point out three general extremes of language performance which can be observed. Most children will show some combination of two or more of these dimensions. The important point here is that the predominance of one of these three features may dictate a different reason for initiating a language program.

It might appear that the goals for a nonverbal child may be different from those for a child who has good grammar and irrelevant content. As it turns out, the goals are quite similar, i.e., appropriate language. If the language programs are reasonably comprehensive in their influence on language performance, they should be effective for both types of presenting behavior.

In order to obtain some information about the relative effects of the language programs on different autistic children, a pilot project was initiated during a summer camp. The camp was run by persons not directly involved in the language program project. All definitions of children, all testing, and all language training sessions were the responsibility of the camp staff and personnel.[1] Language project staff members assisted in the testing of the children and in the training of the camp tutors in the programmed conditioning procedures.

The test population consisted of eight boys and six girls ranging in age from 6.0 to 11.5 years with a mean of 8.9 years. The children had been classified as autistic and accepted into the program prior to the involvement of any language project staff members. Each child was assigned to one camp counselor who accompanied him throughout his entire day. In addition to language performance problems, the children evidenced other undesirable behaviors such as biting, tantrums, isolation, incontinence, etc., which were worked on during the camp activities.

Three thirty-minute language training sessions were scheduled for each day. The children were seen in groups of from two to five. When not in language training sessions, the children and their counselors engaged in swimming, motor training activities, meals, hikes,

1. The authors would like to gratefully acknowledge the help and assistance of Dr. Robert Bradfield, San Francisco State College, California, who was responsible for the camp, for the use of the language programs in that situation, and for his permission to cite the data in this chapter.

and other camp-associated activities. During the nonlanguage training activities, each counselor encouraged his charge to use the specific language targets that were being sought in class; appropriate language responses were reinforced whenever they occurred.

There were two occasions during the camp when language samples were taken. One sample was obtained during the first week of camp and a second was taken one month later during the last week of camp. Both examples were obtained on each child individually in situations that were as nearly identical as possible.

Each sample consisted of two parts. The first part was a timed ten-minute period during which a teacher interacted in a free play situation with the child in order to obtain a language sample. All utterances of the subject were recorded in terms of three classifications: vocalizations of single words, phrases, and sentences. In the second part, a different teacher administered a diagnostic sentence test (PCLT).

Based upon the outcome of the initial testing, the children were placed into one of four language classes. Class A consisted of the two youngest; they could be identified as belonging to the first category of autistic language performance, i.e., no noticeable verbal and little nonverbal communication. A considerable amount of time had to be spent on just getting them to attend to the training situation. After this had been accomplished to some degree, the "Identification of Nouns" (No. 1) program was initiated. Following this program the "Naming Nouns" (No. 2) program was started at the level of individual sounds.

On the pretest one child made no verbalizations and the other made only one. Post-test information showed that the mute child made 117 vocalizations and the other child made 125. Neither made any vocalizations which could be classified as phrases or sentences.

Class B included five children. Their pretest language performance was somewhat higher than that of Class A. Children in this class demonstrated some echolalia and some jargon responses along with accurate verbalizations. They averaged 40 verbal responses each on the conversational pretest. Figure 36 presents the distribution of pre- and post-test responses over the categories of PCLT, words, phrases, and sentences. It can be seen that the higher proportion of responses fell in the single word (or vocalization) category; however, there was a noticeable amount of phrase and sentence responses. The programming for this class began with the "Naming Nouns" (No. 2) program and then moved to the "Is" (No. 4) program. Post-test data indicated that the

Figure 36

Mean PCLT Scores and Distribution of Pre- and
Post-Test Responses Over Words, Phrases, and
Sentences for the Five Children in Class B

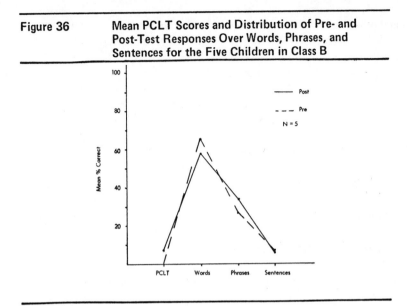

number of verbalizations per child in the conversational sample averaged
80. This was double the amount obtained on the pretest. Again, by
referring to Figure 36, it can be seen that there was a small change in
the distribution of these responses over the various categories. With
double the amount of verbalization, the drop in single word responses
and the increase in phrase responses do take on more meaning than
casual inspection of the graph might otherwise warrant.

The echolalic performance of one child in this group
remained virtually unchanged. Another demonstrated an 80 percent
reduction in echolalic responses while a classmate evidenced a 30 percent increase.

Class C was comprised of three children whose pre-
language performance was higher than either Class A or B. These children tended to have reasonably good language structure and could
communicate fairly well. There was a more pronounced trend toward
echolalia and irrelevant responses within this group than that of either
of the previous ones. Figure 37 shows the pre- and post-test results for
group C. The distribution of verbal responses in the pretest situation is
more heavily weighted towards phrases and sentences than for either of
the two preceding sections. These children had an average of 40 verbal
responses during the pretesting situation. Although their language performance demonstrated the use of *is*, it was decided to begin this group
on the "Is" (No. 4) program. The reasoning was that possibly the high
structure of the program would increase the accuracy of the response as
well as reduce the echolalia.

Figure 37

Mean Pre- and Post-PCLT Scores and Distribution of Spontaneous Language Samples Over Words, Phrases, and Sentences for the Three Children in Class C.

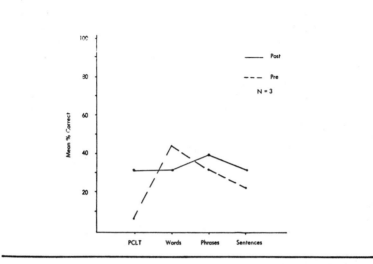

The post-test information indicates that there was no pre-post-difference in the number of verbal responses per child. Figure 37 indicates that there was a shift in responding—away from single words and towards phrases and sentences. Thus, the data suggest some substantial shifting in the quality of verbal responding. As far as echolalia was concerned, one child showed no change, one evidenced complete absence of it, and the other demonstrated a 30 percent increase.

Class D had three children also (one child was dropped because of adequate language performance). Their language was relatively quite good. Figure 38 shows that on the pre-test their distribution of verbal responses over the three categories was equivalent to Class C. However, they scored substantially higher on the PCLT than did Class C. Their average number of verbal responses on the pretest was 37, which was slightly less than that of Class C.

The most noticeable feature of the language of these children was a tendency towards irrelevant content and fantasy type responses. Again, it was decided to begin this class on the "Is" (No. 4) program with the expectation that the structure of the programming would improve overall accuracy of the verbal performance.

Figure 38	Mean Pre- and Post-PCLT Scores and Distribution of Spontaneous Language Samples Over Words, Phrases, and Sentences for the Three Children in Class D.

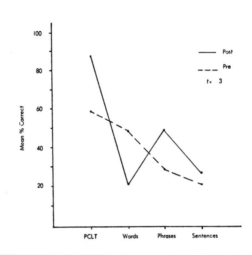

On the post-test sample the average number of verbal responses was 68. Figure 38 indicates that there was a considerable shift in the proportion of verbalizations falling into the word and phrase categories. The PCLT score of 90 indicates that accuracy as well as verbal performance was approaching adequate levels.

Considering the entire group of children, the mean number of verbal responses emitted during the testing situation increased from 37 to 68. This was significant beyond the $p = .01$ level ($t = 4.298/df = 12$). The other changes which can be seen on the graphs are not statistically significant; however, the trend across classes towards more complex language usage is very noticeable. Since this particular project did not include a control group, no hard conclusions can be put forth. Yet there is useful information to be gained from this experience.

Effect upon the echolalic response was very uneven. Some children would show a marked reduction while others would show an increment. We could derive no information from this data which would help us explain either circumstance.

The most noticeable and dramatic change was in Class A because these children went from virtually mute to vocal children. On the other hand, the change in Classes B, C, and D was more subtle but very important in terms of response complexity.

Mentally Retarded Children. Our experience with moderately and severely mentally retarded children is quite promising. With the trainable mentally retarded population (IQ≤50), we have programming experience with 111 children. Most of this is on the earlier programs. Generally we have found that program accuracy remains about the same, and the number of responses to complete a program (and thus program run time) is roughly doubled. For the sequence of "Naming Nouns" (No. 2), "In/On" (No. 3), and "Is" (No. 4) the average accuracy is 80.5 percent with σ 17.7 and the average number of responses to completion is 533 with σ 113.9. Our data for 17 TMR children who have been through the same sequence is accuracy = 82.1 percent with σ 8.9 and responses to completion = 944 with σ 118. However, we do not have sufficient information at this time to indicate how far through the curriculum a TMR child can be expected to progress—this will most likely vary considerably from child to child.

Deaf Children. Obviously, the language programs as presented in this book would be of questionable value to a child who has no usable hearing. To make these programs appropriate for such a child, certain topographical changes would have to be made in order to make up for the loss of auditory input. These changes can include speech reading, signing, finger spelling, or a cued speech type of presentation which combines aspects of signing and finger spelling.

Two such methods are called Cued Speech (Cornett, 1967) and Seeing Essential English (See). These types of signing differ from other procedures in two major respects. First, traditional signing procedures communicate by means of ideas or concepts. Thus, the word "light" might have seven different signs—each one corresponding to a particular definition of the word. In these two methods, as in regular English, each word has only one sign. Secondly, these methods incorporate special signs for prefixes and suffixes. These methods are transmitting more grammatic information than the traditional procedures.

These two characteristics of the Cued Speech and the See methods mean that they are representing English language and grammatic rules rather than ideas and concepts. By using either of these methods of visual stimulus support in conjunction with the language program, we have found it possible to teach language to deaf children.

Using this combined approach the teacher establishes the protocol of programmed conditioning and uses the Cued Speech or See method for the first portion of each program. Then the teacher begins to fade out the visual cueing until finally both teacher and child are working on the program without any cueing by either of them. The most difficult problem has been in establishing the protocol and occasionally the initial program response. Frequently we have had to use auxiliary instructions. Once these two things have been acquired the program run data for deaf children are commensurate with run data from hearing children.

Seven male and eight female students ranging in age from 12.8 to 16.7 years with a mean age of 14.7 years were classified by 1964 ISO standards as having either severe or profound hearing losses. Ten of them went through the "Is" (No. 4) program and five went through the "Is Verbing" (No. 5) program. The pooled data for the fifteen students yielded the following results. The mean precriterion test, which was administered with signs, was 37.3 percent. The mean post-criterion test, which was administered without signs, was 100 percent. It took an average of 3.7 hours to complete a program with signing being discontinued at 2.4 hours.

There was no configuration noted in the data which made them remarkable from previously reported results for hearing students; the information reported here is equivalent to that for other deaf students. For the deaf students, the change in performance was improved grammatic language structure. The language training did not affect the prosody or tonality of their speech.

Although our experience in this areas has not been extensive, the results obtained with this combined procedure by teachers of the deaf have been uniformly encouraging. With some topographical adjustments (a visual support system), the language programs appear to be functionally operational and appropriate for the language nonuser who is profoundly deaf.[1]

Hard of Hearing Children. The child who has some usable hearing is in a different situation from the deaf child. So long as a child can receive the auditory portion of the programs there is no reason to suggest a different kind of teaching method. If amplification will augment the hearing, it should be used. In either case, the teaching goal is the same. The teacher will have to make individual judgments about the appropriateness of permitting the child (or in some cases requiring him) to use speech reading to supplement his ability to hear and receive spoken messages. This decision should be made early in the programming and used consistently throughout as an integral part of the program.

We have had the opportunity to see hard of hearing children in our language programs. In all cases they have been included

1. The authors would like to acknowledge Miss Gretchen Estok of the Los Angeles County School System for her assistance in working with the deaf and for permission to cite the data in this chapter.

in the regular clinical routine of the Clinical Services Department at the Behavioral Sciences Institute. Thus, a hard of hearing child might be grouped with two or three other nonlanguage normal hearing users for group language training. The only feature which might permit an observer to identify the child as hard of hearing would be the presence of a hearing aid or an auditory trainer. During the four years we have been monitoring the language programs, we have had from one to four hard of hearing children receiving language training at any one time. Although the total number of hard of hearing children seen is not large, approximately ten in four years, there has usually been at least one enrolled at all times.

The single performance characteristic which distinguishes these children is that it takes more run time for them to complete a program; one which is usually completed in two hours of run time may go four to five hours with a hard of hearing child. This is especially marked in the beginning and becomes less pronounced later. With the exception of this one factor, we have not been able to identify any differences in the performance data of these children which would distinguish them from the general population of children who have been on the program.

English as a Second Language

The children who speak a language other than English have particular problems communicating. The have difficulty understanding what is said to them as well as being understood by others. These are often called bilingual children. The problem in fact is that they are not bilingual. If they are to successfully survive in education, as well as in their new life environment, they must learn the new language.

The one advantage for them over nonlanguage children is that they already have a functioning language performance. The task is still to teach the English language system and that involves grammar as well as content. Therefore, it might be hypothesized that the language programs would be just as appropriate for them as for nonlanguage children. The reasoning here is that the programs were originally written for children with no language at all. Since non-English speaking children already have a language performance, the task may become more one of conversion rather than original acquisition.

In an effort to compare the results between obtained data on nonlanguage children and non-English speaking children, two separate projects were initiated with normal Spanish speaking, non-

English speaking children. These two projects were 400 miles apart[1] and were not specifically associated with each other. Each of them was developed independently and had its own staff of teachers and its own protocol. The two areas that the projects did have in common were: (1) training of seven-year-old Spanish-speaking children and (2) usage of the language programs. The only involvement of the language project staff was in training the teachers and making one on-site visit to each project; testing and the teaching decisions were made and carried out independently in each group.

One project had seven boys and eighteen girls with a group mean age of 7.4 years. The children were seen in groups of three to four for 30-minute lessons over 23 days. Following the language training sessions, the students were involved in a more omnibus language-usage-experience session for another 30-minute period.

The other project had eight boys and five girls with a mean age of 6.1 years. These children were seen in groups of two for 30-minute periods over a calendar time equivalent to the other project. In this project there were four teachers who had only minimal training in the running of the language programs. The children had no additional scheduled language training session.

Testing preceded and followed the training for both groups of children. Both projects yielded increments in NSST scores for receptive and expressive abilities. As might be anticipated from the descriptions, the project with the two well-trained teachers and the additional language practice class produced results that were noticeably higher than the results of the other project. Figure 39 presents the pooled data for both projects on NSST scores by age equivalent and by raw score. In addition to these findings of a quite substantial increment in language test performance, there were other interesting results. In the first project the teachers gave, in addition to the language tests, a Draw-A-Person test. The before and after age equivalent went from 4.7 years on the before test to 6.2 years on the after test. This difference was statistically significant beyond the p = .01 level of confidence with $t = 3.95/df = 22$. It would be very difficult to argue that the language training program increased maturation or intelligence by such an amount in so brief a time. A more reasonable speculation is that this "non-language biased test" is in fact sensitive to the degree of environmentally appropriate language ability of the test taker. The increment in

1. The authors would like to gratefully acknowledge Mrs. Pat LaBerge, San Jose State College, California, and Mr. Robert Christensen, Goleta Unified School District, California, directors of the two projects with Spanish children, for their assistance and cooperation during their respective projects and for permission to cite the data in this chapter.

154

Figure 39   Mean Pre- and Post-NSST Receptive and Expressive Scores in Language Age (Years) for the Pooled Data from Two Different Projects for Normal Spanish Speaking (Non-English Speaking) Children

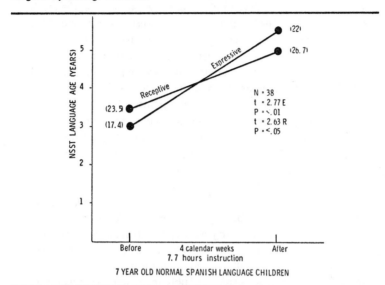

7 YEAR OLD NORMAL SPANISH LANGUAGE CHILDREN

NSST expressive scores also was significant beyond the p = .01 level, with t = 4.009/df = 24 where p @ .05 = t = 2.01.

The other project yielded more modest gains in both expressive and receptive test performance with neither increment reaching significance at the p @ .05 level. However, the teachers gave an additional test, the Englemann Concept Inventory test, Level 1, (Englemann, 1967), to this group. The increment in the post-test score approximated significance at the p = .05 level with t = 2.045/df = 12 where p @ .05 = t = 2.064. As in the other case, this increment probably does not reflect any attribute of the language programs as much as it does the sensitivity of the test to the taker's environmentally appropriate language ability.

These side issues of the Draw-A-Person and Englemann tests do have important bearing upon the language programs. They reflect the breadth of impact that appropriate performance has in the measurement tools commonly used. The results of these two tests also help support the observation that the language programs result in a wide range of impact. The high structure and specificity of the programming procedure does not necessarily preordain that the resultant effects also must be narrow and highly specific. If the mini-language concept is to be valid, then transfer of training and generalization must occur over a substantial range of language related activities.

Although these two language projects were rather brief in duration and were run during school vacation time, the results are quite promising. The programs ran at an average accuracy of 90 percent correct responding. The teachers found that they could skip (using placement procedures) 60 percent of the steps in a typical 25-step program. This plus the run data as well as the pre- and post-results suggest that these procedures are appropriate for use in teaching English as a second language. This experience also points up the desirability of a language usage practice time in addition to programming. This is probably more relevant for non-English speaking children because they do not usually hear English or have an opportunity to consistently speak it at home. The absence of the practice period in the second project probably accounted for the smaller gains in test scores.

One of the more optimal procedures to teach English as a second language might be to give grammatic information in small bursts (programmed conditioning lessons) and then spend an equal or greater amount of time in language usage practice activities. The high probability that the child will have no opportunity to speak English at home makes these practice sessions doubly important. To become a proficient user of the language the child must be able to practice using it. If his home environment does not provide that opportunity, the overall language training strategy must provide for it.

Teacher-Aides

In previous chapters there was considerable discussion about training aides, subprofessionals, or volunteers to carry out the programs. An immediate thought which comes to mind when this topic is raised is whether or not an aide can carry out the programs with the same level of accuracy and efficiency as a professional teacher. The Children's House setting gave us a very good opportunity to explore that very critical question.

Under normal operating conditions, each three-hour session of Children's House was staffed by one professional teacher and two trained aides. Twenty aides were needed each week to provide an appropriate environment for comparing teacher-aide activity. Aides engaged in the same teaching activities as did the teacher except that few of them ever ran the show and tell sessions or the entire group of seven children; more than likely the group size was restricted to a maximum of three or four.

During a series of 51 consecutive language training sessions careful records were obtained concerning whether the person giving the program was an aide or the teacher. In addition, data were collected concerning percent correct responding of the children and total number of responses per child per session. The results indicated that there was no difference between the accuracy levels obtained by the teacher and by the aides; however, the teacher's response rate per child was 28 percent higher than that reported for sessions run by volunteers.

Results indicate that there is no drop in the accuracy of the child's responses because he is working with a trained teacher-aide rather than a teacher. Of course, it must be emphasized that the teacher-aides were trained and experienced. The lower response rate for teacher-aides is not unexpected in view of the setting of Children's House. Most of the teacher-aides worked for one session per week which means that they were there for only three and one-half hours per week. Of that time, about 45 minutes was spent by them in actual programming. With this in mind, it would appear reasonable to anticipate that the response rate would be less for teacher-aides due to lack of practice. Proficiency and speed of any task are usually improved with continued usage. The relatively low level exposure of the volunteers to programming activities could be considered to contribute significantly to the response rate. This suggestion is further substantiated by the observation that those aides who work more frequently than once a week generate response rates that approximate those of the teacher. Also, these teacher-aides are able to conduct show and tell as well as the large (six to seven) group sessions. This, no doubt, also is due to the amount of work time and personal facility with the procedures.

Run Data

The term "run data" has been used and defined throughout this book. They are the on-line operational characteristics of a program used across teachers and students. Run data provides information concerning the performance expectations of students who are on a given program. If a student's run data on a program are within the values given in the run data for the program, the teacher can be reasonably confident that the student's terminal behavior will be equivalent to that reported for the program. Good run data are no guarantee of success, but they do provide on-line information concerning the likelihood of success.

There are seven different categories of information which are included in the run data (see Table 13). The first two are percent correct responding and the σ. This information gives the accuracy level of student performance on the program. The next two items are the number of responses needed to complete the program and the associated σ. These data yield information concerning the total number of responses that the student will have to make, on the average, to complete the program. The fifth category is the time, in program run hours, that is needed to complete the program. The last two pieces of information are usually grouped together for comparative purposes. These are the percent correct responding of the student on the criterion test given prior to the administration of the program and the percent correct responding on the criterion test given after completion of the program. This information provides one measure of the change in target performance that was effected by the program.

During the development of the programs, certain steps were taken to provide a frame of reference for the run data. Run data were obtained exclusively from the training operations of Children's House and the Clinical Services Department of the Behavioral Sciences Institute. Teachers in these two environments were under frequent observation and also held weekly meetings with the project staff to review the performance of each child. Very rigid constraints were placed upon the teacher's administration of the program. No variance from the given protocol was permitted due to the necessity of testing the programs completely.

Other factors went into the characteristic of the run data. One being the fact that new teachers and aides were continually being trained at the two training locations; run data were collected only on totally run programs. Otherwise, placement procedures in later programs would reduce the size of the entries under the response and time categories. Finally, run time was figured on a fractional basis in group sessions. That is, six students seen for one hour would be computed at ten minutes per student; thus, the run data reported for the language programs should be viewed as conservative figures. The run data should be looked upon as the lowest expected values. As an example, off-site locations which reported back data on the programs showed an accuracy score for the "Is" (No. 4) program which was ten percentage points higher than that which is reported in the run data.

Run data will be presented for the grand total of all programs which were completely run as well as for each individual program in the core group. Run data on the other individual programs are not presented here due to their equivalence and redundancy. This information is presented in Table 13.

Our experience has been that, occasionally, students will run through a program at an accuracy level ranging in the high 70's

Table 13   Program Run Data

Program	% Correct	σ	No. Responses	σ	Time	Criterion % Before	Test % After
All Programs	89.9*	16.1	794.0	102.0	3.7	22.0	93.0
Core Programs							
1 Identification of Nouns	80.4	13.3	666.0	55.5	2.5	33.0	100.0
2 Naming Nouns	69.3	33.0		78.5	2.3	0.0	100.0
3 In/On	92.3	12.1	446.0	18.1	1.8	12.5	90.0
4 Is	80.0	6.2	639.0	245.0	3.0	3.9	92.4
5 Is Verbing	90.2	6.9	631.8	296.0	1.8	2.5	96.9
6 Is Interrogative	93.9	5.2	586.3	16.0	2.2	0.0	87.1
7 What Is	92.0	13.6	742.5	18.3	3.5	24.0	92.8
8 He/She/It	87.8	12.0	1064.0	522.0	2.0	22.8	84.0
9 I am	95.0	4.6	665.0	32.6	2.6	29.0	97.0
10 Singular Noun Present Tense	78.3	15.9	1502.0	30.6	6.6	16.0	88.0
11 Plural Nouns Present Tense	77.9	16.5	1377.0	38.3	7.1	20.0	89.4
12 Cumulative Plural/Singular Present Tense	81.8	10.8	1725.0	37.0	6.0	20.0	80.0
13 The	88.0	13.7	836.0	36.5	3.9	67.3	92.5

*All scores are in mean values.

or low 80's. When they complete the program, the criterion test measure and the observation of spontaneous language indicate that they do have and use the language target performance. Students who perform on a program at an accuracy level of between 40 and 60 percent correct usually will not successfully complete the program. Thus, it appears that the current programs are running somewhat above the minimum value needed for successful acquisition of the target.

Summary

We have, in this chapter, tried to present results with a wide variety of children classified according to traditional labeling procedures. This group of categories was not meant to be inclusive nor exclusive of other children. Rather, it was meant to give some perspective to the idea that the teaching task is the same in most cases of language nonusers.

The data presented in this chapter should not be taken as proof of anything. They should be viewed as a report of the experience of a variety of teachers and children who were using Programmed Conditioning for Language Training. To the casual observer, it may appear as if an attempt were being made to present a single procedure to answer all of the "different" language problems. This is not the case. Rather, all of the "groups" of children presented in this chapter are seen as belonging to only one group in terms of a language teaching strategy. They are all expressive, oral language nonusers. The original cause of their nonlanguage performance may differ from child to child. This does not alter the fact that the same universal programs may be appropriate for training expressive, oral language performance in all nonusers.

References

Cornett, R. Oralism vs. manualism: Cued speech may be the answer. *Hearing and Speech News,* 1967, *35,* 6-9.

Dunn, L. M. *Peabody picture vocabulary test.* Minneapolis: American Guidance Service, 1959.

Englemann, S. *The basic concept inventory: Field research edition.* Chicago: Follett Educational Corporation, 1967.

Fygetakis, L. and Gray, B. Programmed conditioning of linguistic competence. *Behaviour Research and Therapy,* 1970, *8,* 153-163.

Goodenough, F. L. *The measurement of intelligence by drawings.* Yonkers-on-Hudson: World Book, 1926.

Gray, B. Language acquisition through programmed conditioning. In R. Bradfield (Ed.), *Behavior modification: The human effort.* San Rafael: Dimensions Press, 1970.

Gray, B. and Fygetakis, L. Mediated language acquisition for dysphasic children. *Behaviour Research and Therapy,* 1968a, *6,* 263-280.

Gray, B. and Fygetakis, L. The development of language as a function of programmed conditioning. *Behaviour Research and Therapy,* 1968b, *6,* 455-460.

Kirk, S., McCarthy, J., and Kirk, W. *Illinois test of psycholinguistic abilities.* Urbana: University of Illinois Press, 1968.

Lee, L. A screening test for syntax development. *Journal of Speech and Hearing Disorders,* 1970, *35,* 103-112.

Ryan, B. and Gray, B. The analysis of certain environmentally generated language samples of linguistically divergent children. Paper presented at American Speech and Hearing Association convention, Chicago, 1971.

Sidman, M. *Tactics of scientific research.* New York: Basic Books, 1960.

Terman, L. and Merrill, M. *Stanford-Binet intelligence scale*, 3rd. rev. Boston: Houghton Mifflin, 1960.

Weschler, D. *Weschler intelligence scale for children.* New York: The Psychological Corporation, 1949.

5 A Behavioral View of Language

Language as a Learned Performance

Several disciplines have become involved in the area of language; they include psychology, education, linguistics, speech pathology, psycholinguistics, and semantics. Generally speaking, linguistics and psycholinguistics are particularly concerned with the *development* and *structure* of language, while psychology (particularly the behavioral group), education, and speech pathology have a greater concern for *methods of teaching* language.

Occasionally these two orientations come into some disagreement with each other over issues of mutual concern. Historically, one of the most active areas of interest is that of normal development of language. This area has been of critical importance in the formulation of linguistic theory as well as in the development of instructional strategy.

With regard to the topic of language acquisition, many linguists in their effort to substantiate the theory of innate capacity for language have said that the Language Acquisition Device (LAD) was responsible for language. Unfortunately, neither the label nor the theory have been put forth in a manner which is scientifically testable. Being untestable, the validity of the idea cannot be confirmed as its supporters rely on circumstantial evidence and verbal persuasion to establish their positions.

A second position is taken by many behaviorists. Behavioral psychology states that each language response must be learned. This S-R theory has been widely discounted by linguists because of the unmanageable proportions that would result if each and every utterance were the result of specific and unique conditioning. Admittedly the characterization of these two positions is polar. But the question still remains, is the development of normal language the result of some innate capacity of the organism or is it the result of learning? As Fodor (1966), we don't feel that either extreme is a satisfactory answer. Unlike Fodor, we do not consider principles of learning to be "simply useless" (p. 112).

To clarify our position on this topic, we would like to begin by presenting some statements by Fodor (1966) in which he discusses the credibility of learning procedures as they relate to language and the concept of base structure.

> . . . by definition, the base structures of a language are not themselves possible utterances in the language. Since. . . base forms are not uttered by children either in operant babbling or at any other stage of verbalization, the desired behavior is not available for selective reinforcement. Hence, in the case of the learning of the base structure of a language, the essential prerequisite for operant conditioning is not satisfied.
>
> In short, a problem that is central to understanding the learning of syntax is that of arriving at a theory of how the child determines the appropriate base structures for the types of sentences that appear in his corpus. However, the peculiarly abstract relation between base structures and sentences unfits any of the usual learning mechanisms for explaining their assimilation (pp. 112-113).

As we interpret these comments, the author appears to discuss the relationship of three entities: (1) base structure (a theoretical construct); (2) children's utterances (an observed performance); and (3) the necessary elements for learning (a behavioral law). The main thrust of the argument is that since the performance of the speaker does not evidence the theoretical construct and since the speaker's performance does not demonstrate the essentials necessary for learning the theoretical construct; therefore, the theoretical construct is validated and the behavioral law is inadequate. This would appear to be a unique conclusion since in most scientific thinking theoretical constructs are validated by the appearance of supporting evidence rather than by the lack of it. Although thoughtful people may be unaccustomed to this type of reasoning, this position is generally representative of many linguists and psycholinguists (McNeill, 1966; Jacobovits and Miron, 1967; Dixon and Horton, 1968).

From our point of view a speaker must hear (or see)

and "learn" each grammar rule. By that we do not mean that he must be able to say the rule or discuss the rule. Rather we mean that the speaker, through his language performance, should demonstrate the use of a rule by its constraint upon his word usage. The grammar rule, or constraint of usage, is a template of linguistic organization which is defined by the observation of specified consistency in the language performance of the speaker. Each word from the corpus must be obtained through learning and assigned to the appropriate grammatic class in which it can appear. To our knowledge, there is no reported evidence of a speaker using either a word from the language corpus of the listener that the speaker never has been exposed to or a correct and unique grammar form that he has not ever seen or heard.[1] On the other hand, there is considerable evidence that potential speakers who have not been exposed to the language don't naturally develop either the words or the grammar. Popular examples include children raised with animals, deaf persons, and foreign speakers. Thus, we are not persuaded by the argument of the linguists. Rather, we find a different point of view to be more plausible, scientifically testable, and in agreement with observed phenomena in the natural environment.

A Fictitious Model of Language

We would like to suggest that the language learning task may not be such an unmanageable thing as it is frequently considered to be. Berger (1968) took samples of conversation from a general adult population until he had a corpus of 25,000 words. From this body, he reported that there were only 2,418 different sentences and 2,507 different words. Half the number of different words was made of single occurrence words. His analysis indicated further that 25,000 words were sufficient to account for all but the rarer ones used in conversation. It would appear that the actual use of the language is not quite as exotic and wide ranging as some have thought it to be. In actuality, our speaking performance appears to be restricted to a relatively few high frequency words and sentences in addition to a large number of very low frequency items.

If we presume that a speaker has a finite number of words available for use, and if we presume that there is a finite set of grammatic usages for those words, then the learning task—while still highly complex—is not overwhelming. A very few words and a limited

---

1. We would not consider the use of seven adjectives to modify one noun or any similar repetitive string as unique. Rather, this would be merely the redundant use of a familiar form. The test would be for the speaker to use just one adjective, if he had never been exposed to adjectives (or the adjective rule) before.

number of grammatic options can result in a language topography which is quite large and which has the appearance of much higher complexity than actually exists. At the risk of being reductionistic, we would like to illustrate this point with an example. The example is quite simplistic and is not a model of actual English performance; however, it does point up the fact that when two separate classes of rather straightforward rules (corpus and grammar) are combined, the result can be geometric with the final topography appearing highly variable and complex.

Example: We have a corpus of 60 words. There is one grammatical construction which is Noun—Verb—Modifier. The constraints upon the word assignments are that twenty of the words can be used in either the Noun or Modifier class, ten of them can be used as either the Noun or Verb class and ten words are unique to each of the three classes. There are no common words between Verb and Modifier. This might be diagrammed as follows:

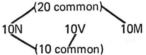

The constraints upon the word sequences are that any Modifier class word may be used with any combination of Noun-Verb. But the Noun-Verb sequence cannot be the same word in both positions, i.e., a common word used twice.

The result of this simple arrangement is that it is possible to generate 23,700 different sequences. If there is an option of using a Modifier and/or a Preposition-the-Noun sequence (which adds three words to the Preposition class and one to the Article class and none to the Noun class), the number of combinations now jumps to 2,844,120 different possible sequences. Obviously, some of the sequences will be propositional and others will be nonsensical. The sorting procedure to eliminate the nonmeaningful sequences is semantics. Thus, word corpus and grammar rules provide the possible sequences and semantic rules provide permissible sequences.

Once again, we would like to emphasize that we are merely highlighting the feasibility of such an arrangement. We are not suggesting that this example is a statement of how it actually occurs. It is interesting to note that with such an uncomplicated example we were able to generate nearly ten times as many sentence sequences as Berger was able to find in a corpus of 25,000 words. It readily can be seen that with more words in the corpus and with more grammar options—such as adding the prepositional phrase—it would be possible to generate a wide, although finite, variety of sequences. Even after semantic screening the remaining chains would still add up to a substantial number.[1]

By learning a set of finite underlying rules of operation, it is possible to generate word *sequences* that are unique in the experience of the speaker. It should be emphasized that only the simultaneous appearance of the specific group of words could be unique. The operating rules which govern the appearance of the group are common and finite rather than unique and infinite. Under this structure, the language learning task becomes more comprehendable and likely.

As an example, word X with its usage, assignments (n,m) could have been learned by a person at some point in time. The usage assignment n could have been acquired initially and then later usage assignment m could have been added. By a similar learning process, the grammar rule *nvm* may have been acquired at a different point in time. If the particular grammar form contained a word usage category (m) that corresponded to one of the assignments (m) for the word X, then there existed the possibility that the two may have occurred together, i.e., *nv* (X m).

If they had occurred together, the speaker would have uttered a sentence that he had not said before. It may be one he never had heard before. The critical point is that once the person had learned the word and the grammar rule—both having a set of mutual constraints—the possibility for their combined occurrence existed. That particular combination may or may not ever have occurred. In either event, both the word and rule had been learned. If uttered, the resultant sentence might have been novel; but all existing elements in it were present in the language performance repertoire of the person prior to its occurrence.

If the language learning task were defined in terms of learning each utterance, then it becomes a highly improbable task. On the other hand, we are suggesting that what must be learned are some words, some rules of assignment, and constraints upon their usage and sequence. When these two sets are combined, their end result is a topography whose complexity belies the learnability of the underlying rules.

---

1. Computer analysis indicated that up to 90% of the sentence types generated would be rational strings.

To us, the terms "competence" or "innate capacity" refer to the ability of the organism to receive, store, process, and sort the language corpus according to a finite number of learned rules of operation.

Some Speculations About Language

In the earlier portions of this book we discussed the mini-language concept. One basic theme was that with a grammatically strong mini-language the child could continue to learn new forms on his own without having to be programmed for them. This would facilitate language acquisition and result in a short training period. Considering the great number of utterances which can be generated from a relatively limited corpus and grammar, it probably would not be functionally necessary for this to occur; however, the ability to self-acquire additional language forms would certainly result in a larger variety of grammatic options for the speaker.

The self-acquiring process must occur in the natural language environment of the speaker. This process would be equivalent to the process used by children who normally acquire language. There, in the environment, he would extract and learn new rules from the examples that bombard him.

The presence of some grammar in the language of the speaker enhances the ease of acquisition of additional grammar. Examples from Chapter Four which point up this observation include the progressive nature of entering language behavior in the transfer of training phenomena and the decreased run time for normal Spanish speaking, non-English speaking children. The finding that for programs of comparable length, later programs run faster than earlier programs lends additional credibility to this position.

Whether it is formally taught or whether it is learned in the natural environment, language is a performance-based skill which requires the learning of a set of rules and a corpus of words. The multiplicative effect of combining grammar rules and the word usage assignment rules is a language topography of tremendous variety.

In order for rule acquisition to occur initially, the speaker must be exposed to the rule through the performance of another speaker in his environment. The point has been made previously that if a speaker is not exposed to the language performance, he will neither acquire nor produce it.

Sequentially, following exposure, the speaker will perform the language according to the rule, revise the rule and its performance, and finally demonstrate correct habitual usage. This usage on the part of the speaker can occur any time following the exposure, or more probably many exposures, of the rule by other speakers in the environment. It must be stressed here that we are talking about the usage of a grammar form anytime following its exposure to the speaker and not the rote imitation of a word chain which has been just previously heard.

In order for the speaker to revise and habitually use the correct form of the rule, his usage of the rule must be heard by and consequated by a listener in his environment. Consequation has two aspects. First, any response to the performance of the speaker by the listener will consequate the performance. This response can be verbal or nonverbal on the part of the listener. The listener can answer a question, reply to a comment, or perform some nonverbal act in response to the performance of the speaker. This listener response will either accelerate or decelerate the probability of future occurrences of the performance on the part of the speaker.

The second aspect of the consequation is the feedback concerning the accuracy of the performance. The listener may, or may not, correct the performance of the speaker and he may, or may not, do this simultaneously while he is responding to the message of the performance as described in the preceding paragraph. Thus, correction on the part of the listener may increase the probability of accuracy in future occurrences of the rule. Therefore, the listener response to a language performance can potentially affect both the frequency of future occurrences of the utterance and also its accuracy.

The correction, by the listener, of inaccurate usages of the rule is not obligatory for revision to occur. A speaker may change his performance based upon his own continued exposure to the proper model; however, the listener's correction could certainly facilitate the revision process of the speaker.

Distinctive grammar forms which are frequently seen in ethnic groups or in particular geographic areas highlight the influence which other speakers and listeners in the environment have on the language performance of the speaker. This phenomenon can be seen also in word usage assignments and articulatory patterns. Such idiosyncratic usages make up a dialect. A dialect is a subset of the language in which its users have persisted in the performance of an "incorrect" rule. This is perpetuated in new speakers (children) through the performance examples of the speakers and the correction process of the listeners.

Speculations can lead far afield, and that is not our purpose. By presenting some speculations and opinions, we have attempted to give the reader a better perspective of the applicability of behavior principles in explaining how language performance occurs. The examples used are not all-encompassing but are quite general. By taking this approach we run the risk of being reductionistic. Alternately, we hope that we have not committed the more grevious error of zealously over-complicating the situation for the sake of having a "complete" answer.

Our goal here is somewhat different. By attempting to explore the credibility of a behavioral explanation of language, in this chapter we describe the mechanisms of language development rather than label them. If they can be successfully explained, the veracity of that description may be put to empirical test. If the data uphold the original premise, they can be retained and used; if not, they can be discarded or modified and retested.

In either event we can avoid the unsolvable morass that some authors have generated for both teachers and researchers alike. The plethora of mystical labels reduces any discussion about language acquisition or structure to an exercise in faith. It is true that one can protect himself from visible error by stating "concepts" in a manner which renders them untestable. This is the main reason for the continued existence of items such as base structure, Language Acquisition Device, innate capacity, etc. Either these and similar labels should be restated in a testable manner, or they should be discarded by those who are genuinely interested in furthering our knowledge and understanding of language and by those who are concerned about developing effective training strategies.

Implications of
the Language Program Experience

In addition to the general contribution of providing language training programs for teaching nonusers to talk, there are other implications of the language program experience.

Receptive Versus Expressive. The programs have focused on oral, expressive language because this has been our target. We assumed that the children with whom we were working were capable of perceiving and processing verbal stimuli, which are the only prerequisites to language training. The programs have demonstrated that expressive language may be taught rather early in the teaching sequence (Program No. 2, Naming Nouns). Apparently, it is not necessary to build an extensive receptive language repertoire using a nonverbal response (pointing, for example) before teaching expressive language. A child may successfully be asked to emit a verbal response early in the teaching sequence. It is possible that the development of an expressive repertoire may actually enhance the learning of a receptive repertoire (Guess, 1969).

Meaning. Although the programs permit semantic variation to occur while appropriate syntactic-grammatical structures are being taught, it has been our observation that children have learned to speak in semantically meaningful sentences. The continuous pairing of pictures, objects, and actions with utterances throughout the programs has undoubtedly contributed a great deal to this outcome. A behavioral index of whether or not a child knew the meaning of a word would be whether or not he uttered the grammatically correct word or words when presented with a stimulus such as a picture, object, action, or question. The ability to define or give the meaning of a word represents another level of semantic proficiency. This latter ability assumes certain basic, expressive language skills on the part of the speaker. By teaching the child a mini-language, we have tried to increase the probability that he can engage in more semantically sophisticated language.

Teaching. The programmed language procedures provide a very clear, concise description of the teaching act. They are teachable, learnable procedures which require only a minimal, circumscribed amount of information by the teacher. They reduce the extensive training period usually required to prepare a teacher. Because they are overt, procedures they can be modified (or expanded easily, if necessary) in a systematic way through branching procedures or through additional programs. The basic program format (delivery system) may be used in teaching many different kinds of behaviors such as reading, arithmetic, and spelling.

Teaching Versus Natural Development. The programs make a contribution to the teaching/learning process. They call attention to the teaching model as an alternative to the developmental model. Historically, interest has been focused on either the language corpus of adult speakers or on the developmental fragments of language of children as they gradually accumulated the adult corpus. The language of children has been studied to determine the developmental milestones and to normalize the appearance of specific phonetic, grammatic, semantic, and syntactic forms. These studies may be described as evaluating the results of natural language teaching. They simply may have been indirectly measuring parental teaching effectiveness rather than any normal, innate developmental process. How else can we explain the wide variations in proficiency found in most skills, in most age groups, in most studies of language development?

Developmental language information, helpful as it may be in determining language content, offers little constructive data on teaching strategies. Even the study of natural teaching methods employed by parents may be of limited value. Many people have learned to swim, play tennis, or read "naturally"; but the learning procedures used in the acquisition of these skills may not be as efficient as those used by the skilled teacher who is following a program. Can we improve on "nature"? By nature we mean the stimuli, responses, and consequences that occur in the child's uncontrolled environment. The answer lies in the careful study of the procedures used by people in the environment to teach children to talk and comparing those to programmed methods. It is possible that environmental teachers (parents) who effectively teach their children to talk are using many of the same procedures, although not so systematically, as found in a language program. In the case of language divergent children, it may be that the parent has inadvertently taught the child "funny" rules of language—or even not to talk.

Emotionally Disturbed Children. The age-old clinical problems of describing the relationship between communicative-emotional difficulty and teaching the emotionally disturbed child have been resolved in a different way. Two classes of behaviors (social behavior and language behavior) have been separated and their interrelationship carefully structured. The "emotionally disturbed" child is first taught to *attend* to the task of learning to speak. He is then taught language. The result generally has been a well-behaved child who speaks appropriately. There may or may not be emotional elements or negative behavior remaining in his repertoire. Some may view this as a form of "psychotherapy." We do not. This is simply a behavioral solution to a common clinical problem. The implication is that emotionally disturbed children may be taught language through a procedure which increases their attention behavior and presents language information in a systematic way.

Readiness. The fact that most of the data on the language programs have been collected on preschool children raises some questions about the "readiness" concept. Readiness is defined as being able to receive, process, and respond to stimuli. The emergence of language in a child only tells the observer that it has been learned. This does not indicate that the child was unable to produce language earlier. Only after careful teaching procedures have produced no language improvement can we be sure that a subject is not physiologically capable or ready. The "onset" of speech may be more contingent upon appropriate teaching strategies and sociological mores than on physiological integrity. Language training may be analagous to toilet training and weaning in that these events are more culturally determined than physiologically prescribed.

Mini-language. The mini-language concept suggests that if basic language forms are taught the child, he eventually will be able to generate appropriate speech on his own. This greatly reduces the teaching burden and also raises questions about the complexity of language. If a child who has been taught a few basic forms can learn the rest by himself, either the organism is extremely capable or the language training task is not as difficult as many would have us believe. Probably both are true. We know very little about the complexity of everyday language. Although the average adult speaker can create extremely complex sentences, does he commonly do so? Or are the sentences he uses really that complicated? This is not to suggest that we think language is a simple skill. We do not think it is. But we wonder if language learning has not been made overly complex by awkward, inappropriate methods of study.

Programming. The programmer's approach to language training has implications. Commonly, the programming process starts with a description of the goal or target response eventually desired. We have defined it as spontaneous language or the ability to generate novel sentences which are grammatically accurate and semantically appropriate. The programmer then works backwards carefully describing each skill, or in this case, language form, which the child must have in order to become a novel sentence generator. The programmer, by necessity, must limit the information he can teach or program. Hopefully, he isolates the critical events such as nouns, verbs, responses to questions, novel responses, etc.

Even if all the rules of language were known, the language programmer would use behavioral indices (usually oral expressive responses) to permit him to judge whether or not a child knew the rule. The ability to verbalize rules is seen as secondary. It only is necessary when educational situations demand that the speaker describe the rules he uses to speak.

Programming brings a certain discipline to the study of language teaching which results in effective teaching programs. The rules of programming serve to separate the functional from the non-functional in terms of delineating the skills one must have to speak. Programming arranges them in a logical, teachable sequence. The programmer is forced to carefully measure his program and its results. This produces reliable, tested, replicable procedures which can be applied by others to teach other children.

The programmer is often dependent upon others to provide the content of that which he will program or teach. He generally seeks out content experts who, in the case of language teaching, are linguists or psycholinguists. They can describe the content of language or what is to be learned. The content of programs in this book was derived from the work of the linguists and the psycholinguists although few of them have assisted directly in the preparation of a program. There is a great opportunity for the content experts (linguists) and the programmers (behaviorists) to work cooperatively in the development of effective, efficient language teaching programs. The only requirement is a mutual respect for each other's information, expertise, and interests. We can only hope that the language programs in this book will encourage more direct cooperation between the two disciplines.

Universal Programs. We attempted to develop universal programs which could be employed with all types of nonusers because universal programs have certain inherent values. First, it now becomes unnecessary to generate a new set of programs for each child. Second, each language teacher does not have to develop his or her own set of programs. This will save hours of needless labor. Third, the skills necessary for program writing and development are quite different from those required for program execution. To enable each teacher to adequately prepare programs would require additional specialized training involving an extensive time commitment. Fourth, the use of a standard program results in a common language among teachers and researchers which promotes a more efficient interchange of ideas and results. Additional procedures which may be necessary for some subgroups of nonusers (autistic children, for example) can be uniformly added in the form of branch sequences, new series, or even new programs. This information can be readily disseminated. An amount of data may be collected and collated on one procedure rather than on several related procedures. This should provide for a more uniform, effective program in a shorter amount of time. And finally, in today's mobile society, standard programs make it possible for children to move around the country and still be able to continue in a systematic, efficient, meaningful language training procedure.

A universal program may be put to other uses. It may be administered as part of an evaluative (diagnostic) battery of procedures which will yield specific information about the learning ability or disability of a given child. The programs also may be used as a tool to study other phenomena such as group versus individual training, optimal training periods, the emergence of various transformations, etc. In short, the programs become a standardized procedure with which other variables may be observed and measured.

Aides and Parents. Finally, the contribution of a programmed, effective procedure which can be carried out by trained aides is not to be minimized. By having several para-professionals carry out systematic procedures under the supervision of a professional teacher, it is possible to extend the teaching service to many more children. A natural evolution of the language programs could be a simplified guide to parents describing how they may teach their children to talk. We have not explored this area extensively because we wanted to control the input of language training to the children, but we visualize that it will be possible sometime in the future to train parents to teach their own children. Perhaps the eventual teaching program model will be extensive classes to teach parents of language divergent children how to teach their own children.

Future Research

The language programs represent a stage of development in the attainment of the goal of effective, efficient training programs. They are functional prototypes of those programs which will follow in the future. The information about programming and language will continue to change and grow. This will be reflected in the programs of the future. Fortunately, the present programs are open ended and new information can be put into them with minimal revision of the basic protocol. More research is needed in both the delivery system (programming) and the content area (language). Rather than try to generate an exhaustive list of research activities, we have chosen to present two examples—one in programming and one in language—to serve as models of the kinds of research for which we see great need.

The first, in the area of programming, concerns computer simulation of training programs. The present strategy is to write a program, test it, revise it, retest it, etc. on actual subjects. This is not only extremely hard work, but it is very time consuming. Computer simulation can provide for the hypothetical testing of training programs in a relatively short period of time. Once a computer program for simulation of student responding is written and developed, it may be used over and over again with different language training variables being tested each time. We undertook such a computer simulation project recently. We developed some information about the abilities of prospective students, description of a training program, the criterion levels desired, and the output test performance expected at the conclusion of the training programs. Most of this information was based on observations of students in training and previous program run data. This information was translated into computer language and computer simulation of program execution was developed.

We are presently exploring the variable of task difficulty to determine the interaction between it and the incoming capacity of students. This kind of programming research should eventually yield much vital information about program construction. It should permit us, a priori, to design a program which will have a high probability of success before it is tested on students.

The second research need, in the area of language, concerns the frequency of the occurrence of various grammatical forms in normal adult language. Very little work has been done in this area. This information is vital to the selection of content for language programs. The frequency of occurrence of various grammatical forms is possibly related to the complexity of their structure. Knowledge of the relative frequency of occurrence of various language forms could help us select those forms to be taught. This would encourage people to focus on a careful description of a circumscribed set of common forms rather than to try to explain all language occurrences. How complex, grammatically speaking, is everyday adult speech? A frequency analysis might be helpful to answer this question. This is the language which the child constantly hears and is the corpus from which he must select his "rules" and usable forms. We have just begun to explore this area, and our major finding so far is that we need a category, or classification system, which will aid us in quickly identifying various grammatical forms from a corpus. A gross system would include present, past, and future; singular versus plural; regular versus irregular verbs; pronouns versus nouns; etc. It is this type of research in language which will help us accurately describe expressive oral language so that we may clearly define the final target behavior of any language teaching program.

Summary

We have attempted to present our theory, our programs, our data, and speculate about language and the teaching of language to nonusers. Our goal has been to describe our procedures so that they may be easily shared with others. As our educational problems become more complex, it behooves all of us to become more effective and accurate in our analysis and treatment of them.

References

Berger, K. The most common words used in conversations. *Journal of Communicative Disorders,* 1968, *1,* 201-214.

Dixon, T. and Horton, D. (Eds.) *Verbal behavior and general behavior therapy.* Englewood Cliffs, N. J.: Prentice-Hall, 1968.

Fodor, J. A. How to learn to talk: Some simple ways. In F. Smith and G. Miller (Eds.), *The genesis of language.* Cambridge: M.I.T. Press, 1966.

Guess, D. A functional analysis of receptive language and productive speech: Acquisition of the plural morpheme. *Journal of Applied Behavior Analysis,* 1969, *2,* 55-64.

Jakobovits, L. and Miron, M. (Eds.). *Readings in the psychology of language.* Englewood Cliffs, N. J.: Prentice-Hall, 1967.

McNeill, D. Developmental psycholinguistics. In F. Smith and G. Miller (Eds.), *The genesis of language.* Cambridge: M.I.T. Press, 1966.

Author Index

Subject Index